Piriformis Syndrome

K. Mohan Iyer

Editor

Piriformis Syndrome

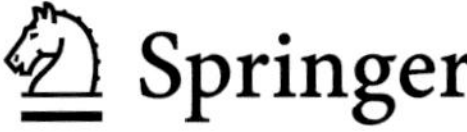 Springer

Editor
K. Mohan Iyer
Retired Consultant Orthopaedic Surgeon
Bengaluru, Karnataka, India

ISBN 978-3-031-40738-3   ISBN 978-3-031-40736-9 (eBook)
https://doi.org/10.1007/978-3-031-40736-9

This Springer imprint is published by the registered company Springer Nature Switzerland AG
The registered company address is: Gewerbestrasse 11, 6330 Cham, Switzerland

Paper in this product is recyclable.

To the memory of my respected teacher

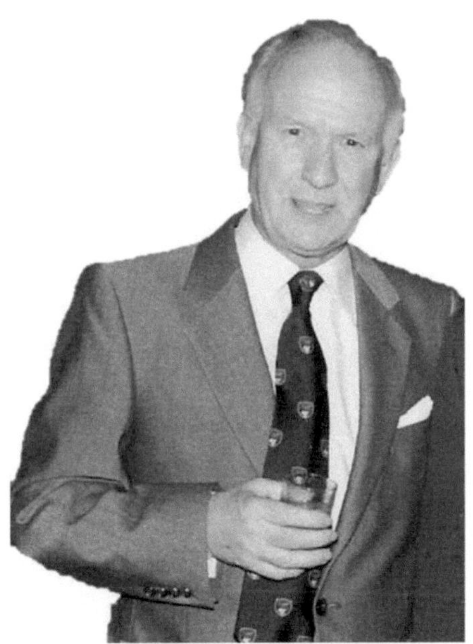

(Late) Mr. Geoffrey V. Osborne

I have written this dedication with a very
heavy mind full of fond memories for my late
respected teacher, Mr. Geoffrey V. Osborne,
without whose constant encouragement and
freedom I could not have written this book.
These teachers are extremely rare to spot

these days where the turmoil of daily life overtakes one's ambitions, duties, and career aspirations. I have a remarkable store of personal and academic memories of him, with whom I spent 4 long years at the University of Liverpool, UK, during which I rarely looked upon him as my teacher, as he was more of a close friend and father to me during all those years.

He inspired me with his approach and knowledge of orthopaedics, that is unforgettable, and I would not have followed his footsteps, had it been for him. I just have hallucinations that he is very much present there and I am sharing with him the joy of being in India. He was a patron of the Indian Orthopedic Association, and he patiently listened when I presented my original research on the Hip Joint, done in Liverpool, with my respected teacher and late Dr. Rasik M. Bhansali who was the chairman at the Conference of the Association of Surgeons of India in December 1982.

and loving thanks to
My Wife, Mrs. Nalini K. Mohan
My Daughter, Deepa Iyer, MBBS, FRCP (UK), FAFRM (RACP)
(1. Honorary Adjunct Assistant Professor/ Bond University, Queensland
2. Senior Lecturer/Griffith University and University of Queensland)
My Son-in-law, Kanishka B.
My Son, Rohit Iyer, BE (IT)
My Daughter-in-law, Deepti B. U.
My Grandsons, Vihaan and Kiaan
My Grandchild, Nisha Iyer.

Foreword

I am delighted to write this foreword for Dr. K. Mohan Iyer's latest book on *Piriformis Syndrome*. My academic association with Dr. Iyer commenced many years ago, when he worked in our hospital on a short assignment. I have subsequently kept in touch with him and have also contributed as an author in some of his previous textbooks. Dr. K. Mohan Iyer has demonstrated a lifelong interest in diseases pertaining to the Hip joint, and this latest book represents an extension of that interest. He has used his knowledge of the anatomy of the Hip joint to good effect by devising a variation of the posterior approach to the Hip in his name. This approach has been cited in various textbooks on the Hip joint and previous editions of Campbell's Operative Orthopaedics.

Piriformis syndrome is a clinical condition, which occurs when the Sciatic nerve is entrapped in the vicinity of the piriformis muscle. This results in symptoms in the ipsilateral buttock and lower limb, which are akin to a lower limb radiculopathy. Making a clinical diagnosis of piriformis syndrome can often times be difficult and is largely based on the history and clinical presentation. The difficulty in making a diagnosis arises due to a lack of specificity and consistency in the clinical tests that are currently available. Patients who present with radicular impingement pain due to lateral recess stenosis or disc pathology may mimic the pain of piriformis syndrome. Special clinical manoeuvres like the Freiberg, Beatty, Pace, and FAIR tests may help to localise the pain in the piriformis area. Patients with symptoms of piriformis syndrome may present to various medical practitioners, both in primary and secondary care settings. In secondary care, these patients can present to Hip, spine and neurosurgical clinics, sports physicians, and doctors with a special interest in the management of chronic pain. They can also present to physiotherapists, occupational therapists, chiropractors, and other allied specialists. This book will, therefore, be of value to a wide range of primary and secondary care physicians, surgeons, and various other allied specialists who deal with Hip and back conditions.

Dr. K. Mohan Iyer and his co-authors should be commended for the time and effort that they have taken in presenting the various aspects of piriformis syndrome, in an easily readable format. These include, but are not restricted to, the anatomy, basic science, aetio-pathology, clinical features, radiology, diagnostics, treatment, and prognosis. The authors have also provided a detailed bibliography at the end of each chapter that the more discerning reader will find helpful.

I am sure that readers of this book will find it a useful source of information in diagnosing and managing piriformis syndrome. I wish the authors success with its publication and am confident that it will be well received by practitioners with an interest in this condition.

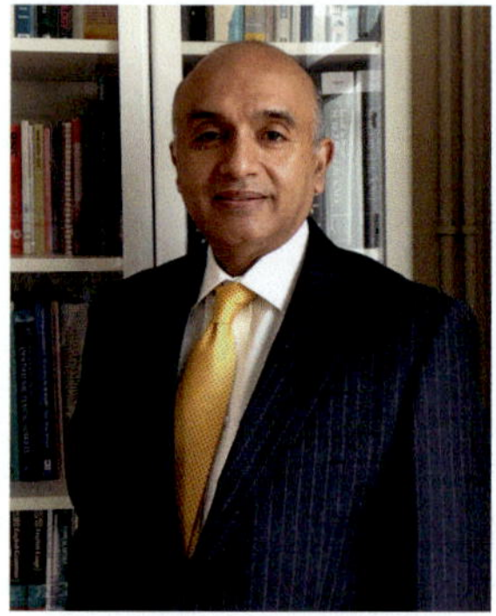

Mr. Dipen K. Menon
MS Orth (AIIMS), MCh (Orth), FRCS
England (Trauma and Orth)

Consultant Trauma and Orthopaedic
Surgeon

Lead Consultant NJR
Lower limb Arthroplasty and Revision
Surgery
BOA Clinical Champion

Director, ATLS Course, Kettering

Kettering General Hospital, NHS
Foundation Trust (Affiliated to
University of Leicester), UK

Preface

The foreword has been given by Mr. Dipen K. Menon, MS (Orth), FRCS (Eng Et Glasg), MCh (Orth), FRCS (Tr Et Orth) Consultant Orthopaedic Surgeon, Kettering General Hospital, NHS Foundation Trust (Affiliated to University of Leicester), UK.

I am extremely thankful to Ahmed Zaghloul, (Lecturer at Orthopaedic Department Mansoura University, Mansoura University Hospitals, Mansoura University, Egypt) along with Ankita Ahuja, (Consultant Radiologist, Innovision Imaging, Mumbai, India), Gaurav Kant Sharma, (Consultant at MSK Radiology, Sports Radiology, and Ultrasound), Karthikeyan. P. Iyengar, (Trauma and Orthopaedic Surgeon, Southport and Ormskirk Hospital NHS Trust, Southport, UK), and Mahmoud Diab Abdelhaleem, (Department of Orthopedic Physical Therapy, Faculty of Physical Therapy, Cairo University, Ahmed El Zaiat St., Bein El Sarayat, Giza 12612, Egypt) for their contribution in the form of chapters for this book Piriformis Syndrome.

My grateful thanks to S. Shanmuga Jayanthan, (Consultant Radiologist, Tanjore, Tamil Nadu), Himanshu Agrawal (Department of Physical Medicine and Rehabilitation, All India Institute of Medical Sciences, Jodhpur, Rajasthan), Mihiro Kaga (Department of Clinical Biostatistics, Graduate School of Medical and Dental Sciences, Tokyo Medical and Dental University, Tokyo, Japan), Ameet Kumar Jha (University of Central Nicaragua, Managua, Nicaragua), Md. Abu Bakar Siddiq (Department of Physical Medicine and Rheumatology, Brahmanbaria Medical College, Brahmanbaria, Bangladesh), Gamze Gül Güleç (İstanbul, Turkey), and Sushumna Tiwarri (Healthcare Management–USA).

I am also thankful to Rajesh Botchu, Consultant Musculoskeletal Radiologist, The Royal Orthopacdic Hospital, Birmingham, UK, for helping me out in Chap. 8.

Above all my grateful thanks to Melisa Morton [Executive Editor Clinical Medicine], Elizabeth Pope and Ram Prasad Chandrasekar for their invaluable help in tis manuscript.

Also my thanks to Vishnu M. G., Project Manager at Straive, Chennai, India for his patience in the production of this book.

Above all, I highly appreciate the help of my son, Mr. Rohit Iyer, in the presentation and publication of this book.

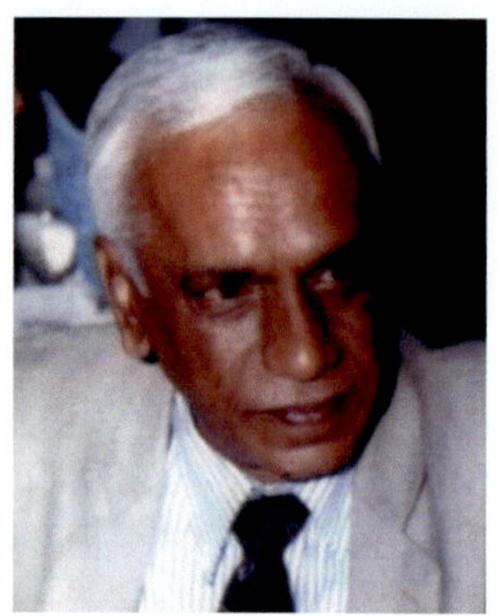

Bengaluru, Karnataka, India

K. Mohan Iyer
MBBS (Mumbai)
MCh Orth. (Liverpool)
MS Orth. (Mumbai)
FCPS Orth. (Mumbai)
D'Orth. (Mumbai)

Contents

Introduction

K. Mohan Iyer

Piriformis syndrome is an uncommon neuromuscular disorder that is caused when the piriformis muscle compresses the sciatic nerve. The piriformis muscle is important in lower body movement because it stabilizes the hip joint and lifts and rotates the thigh away from the body. It enables us to walk, shift our weight from one foot to another, and maintain balance. It is also used in sports which involve lifting and rotating the thighs, in almost every motion of the hips and legs.

LBP [Low back pain] most commonly involves one of the following conditions: sciatic nerve entrapment, herniated nucleus pulposus, direct trauma, muscle spasm due to chronic or overuse injury, or piriformis syndrome.

Piriformis syndrome occurs when this muscle presses on the sciatic nerve (the nerve that goes from the spinal cord to buttocks and down the back of each leg) which can cause pain and numbness in the lower body.

Piriformis syndrome is an uncommon cause of buttock and hip pain due to entrapment of the sciatic nerve by the piriformis muscle at the greater sciatic notch. Entrapment of the sciatic nerve by the piriformis muscle was first described in 1928 by Yeoman. In 1937 Freiberg described such entrapment in great detail, specifying that it can be distinguished from other causes of radicular pain such as disc herniation, extrinsic pressure by tumor or other mass, or intrinsic nerve abnormality. Pace's sign has also been described (pain and weakness in association with resisted abduction and external rotation of the affected thigh. Robinson first introduced the term piriformis syndrome in 1947, and enumerated six classic diagnostic findings:

1. History of trauma to the sacroiliac and gluteal areas.
2. Pain at the sacroiliac joint, greater sciatic notch, and piriformis muscle that radiates down the limb and causes difficulty walking.
3. Acute exacerbation of pain by stooping or lifting and moderate relief of pain by traction in a supine position.

K. Mohan Iyer (✉)
Bangalore, Karnataka 560003, India
e-mail: kmiyer28@hotmail.com

K. M. Iyer (ed.), *Piriformis Syndrome*,
https://doi.org/10.1007/978-3-031-40736-9_1

1

4. Palpable sausage-shaped tender mass over the piriformis muscle on the painful side.
5. Positive Lasegue's sign.
6. Gluteal atrophy, depending upon duration of the affliction.

It is a clinical condition which is believed to be caused by compression of the sciatic nerve by the piriformis muscle. Piriformis syndrome (PS) is a somewhat vague diagnosis marked by lower back, buttock, and upper posterior thigh pain. It can cause pain or numbness in the buttock and down the back of the leg. Piriformis syndrome usually begins with pain, tingling, or numbness in the buttocks. Often symptoms are caused and made worse by sitting or running.

Piriformis syndrome is more common in females by a 6:1 ratio, thought to be due to anatomical differences. In about 20% of the population, the sciatic nerve or some of its branches innervate the piriformis muscle.

The Piriformis muscle is divided into 2 parts by peroneal division of the sciatic nerve going between the 2 parts of the muscle.

There are 2 types of Piriformis Syndrome namely:

(1) Primary Piriformis Syndrome: This type is seen in cases which have a anatomical variation such as a split piriformis muscle or sciatic nerve or a different path of the sciatic nerve. These type are about 15% of cases of Piriformis Syndrome.
(2) Secondary Piriformis Syndrome: This is usually because of some other causes such as trauma giving rise to ischemia.
  a. Nerve compression giving rise to spasms and inflammation of the buttocks.
  b. In Piriformis Syndrome, muscle spasms are usually due to trauma or due to lumbar and sacroiliac joint pathologies.
  c. Altered biomechanics of the lower limb, low back and pelvic regions giving rise to compression may also be the cause of Piriformis Syndrome giving rise to signs and symptoms in other regions of the sciatic nerve such as buttock, leg and feet.
  d. Excessive use of the piriformis muscle such as running may give rise to compression termed as "wallet neuritis" due to repeated trauma due to sitting on hard surfaces.

Most patients complain of acute tenderness in the buttock and sciatica-like pain down the back of the thigh, calf and foot. Typical piriformis syndrome symptoms may include: A dull ache in the buttock or a pain down the back of the thigh, calf and foot similar to sciatica. There is no definitive test for piriformis syndrome. Many cases may give a history of trauma or sitting for longer durations.

The SERS [Short External Rotators] comprising the piriformis muscle (PM), superior gemellus (SG), inferior gemellus (IG), obturator internus (OI), which was a far superior method to the reattachment technique in terms of contiguity and muscle atrophy as seen by a long-term postoperative follow-up using magnetic resonance imaging (MRI).

The piriformis muscle is an important surgical landmark for the posterior approach to the hip as it has a close relationship to the sciatic nerve and to the entry point for the

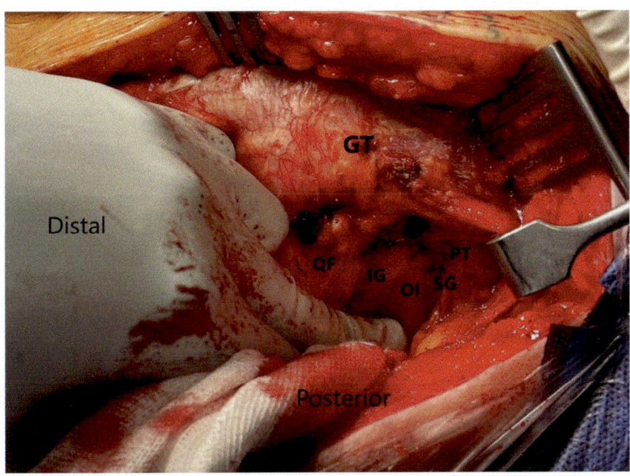

Fig. 1 Short external rotators comprising the piriformis muscle (PT), superior gemellus (SG), inferior gemellus (IG), obturator internus (OI) [Courtesy: Figure reproduced with kind permission of Ahmed Salah El-Din Osman Zaghloul < ahmed_zaghloul@mans.edu.eg]

femoral canal. Many variations in the morphological appearance in piriformis have been described, with the most common one being the belly of piriformis split into upper and lower portions by the sciatic nerve or one of its components. Preservation of the piriformis tendon is far superior to reattachment technique in terms of contiguity and muscle atrophy using magnetic resonance imaging. Piriformis muscle appears to function as a posterior stabilizer of the Hip joint in 90° of flexion and hence leaving the tendon intact appears to decrease the risks of dislocation.

Piriformis syndrome when seen is a peripheral neuritis of the sciatic nerve caused by an abnormal condition of the piriformis muscle and is characterized by hip and buttock pain. Effectively, piriformis syndrome is a form of 'sciatica' caused by compression of the sciatic nerve by the piriformis muscle. Symptoms may include pain on sitting along with pain through the sacrum, gluteal region and thigh or pain with single leg movements with Pain when getting up from sitting or squatting. MRI imaging is highly accurate at assessing both bone and soft tissue pathologies since MRI imaging can accurately demonstrate and measure both the size of the piriformis, size and variation in the sciatic nerve. Diagnostic musculoskeletal ultrasound imaging is ian excellent imaging tool for assessing for soft tissue hip pathology as well as being useful for measuring the size and thickness of structures such as the piriformis muscle and the sciatic nerve. Ultrasound appears to be a reliable technique for the diagnosis of piriformis syndrome (Fig. 1).

It is also known by other names such as Pseudosciatica; Wallet sciatica; Hip socket neuropathy; Pelvic outlet syndrome; Low back pain.

In around 80% of people, the common fibular nerve penetrates the muscle.

Epidemiology of Piriformis Syndrome

K. Mohan Iyer

Piriformis syndrome (PS) is an unusual type of extra-spinal sciatica which is a mixture of conditions around the piriformis muscle (PM) and the adjacent sciatic nerve (SN).

PS may be primary where patients show clinical manifestations that can be elicited by sprcial signs which may show EMG abnormalities, or other causes, where a precipitating event such as trauma or aberrant anatomy, may lead to compression of the sciatic nerve. This has an anatomical cause, with variations such as a split piriformis muscle, split sciatic nerve, or an anomalous sciatic nerve path. Among patients with piriformis syndrome, fewer than 15% of cases have primary causes. At present, there are no accepted values for the prevalence of the anomaly and little evidence to support whether or not the anomaly of the sciatic nerve causes piriformis syndrome or other types of sciatica. These findings suggest that piriformis and sciatic anomalies may not be as important to the pathophysiology of piriformis syndrome as previously thought.

Secondary piriformis syndrome occurs as a result of a precipitating cause, including macrotrauma, microtrauma, ischemic mass effect, and local ischemia. It has the following important features such as:

(1) Nearly half of the cases may by macrotrauma to the buttocks, leading to inflammation of soft tissue, muscle spasms, or both, with resulting nerve compression.
(2) Muscle spasms of the PM are usually caused by direct trauma, post-surgical injury, lumbar and sacroiliac joint pathologies or overuse.
(3) PS may also be caused by shortening of the muscles due to the altered biomechanics of the lower limb, low back and pelvic regions and can result in compression or irritation of the sciatic nerve. Due to a dysfunction of the piriformis muscle, causes various signs and symptoms such as pain in the sciatic nerve

K. Mohan Iyer (✉)
Bangalore, Karnataka 560003, India
e-mail: kmiyer28@hotmail.com

K. M. Iyer (ed.), *Piriformis Syndrome*,
https://doi.org/10.1007/978-3-031-40736-9_2

distribution, including the gluteal area, posterior thigh, posterior leg and lateral aspect of the foot.

(4) Microtrauma may also result from overuse of the piriformis muscle, such as in long-distance walking or running or by direct compression. An example of this kind of direct compression is known as "wallet neuritis", which is a repetitive trauma caused by sitting on hard surfaces.

The common type of PS is an deep gluteal pain which radiates to the ipsilateral thigh, which may be increased by rotation of the hip in flexion or knee extension, along with tenderness over sciatic notch, and atrophy of gluteus maximus. The incidence of Piriformis syndrome ranges from 5 to 36%. PS may lead to pathologic conditions of the sciatic nerve giving rise to sciatic neuropathies also which may be seen as foot drop that may mimic a common fibular neuropathy at the knee, weakness in knee flexion, ankle plantar flexion, ankle inversion with a normal or decreased ankle jerk and pain with sensory loss in the foot; Males are affected more likely to have a tumor and affected females are more likely to have an aberrant anatomy. Steroid injections appear to be seen in most cases with chronic conditions.

Predisposing Factors

K. Mohan Iyer

Piriformis syndrome is a peripheral neuritis that is caused by either hypertrophy, inflammation, or anatomical variation of piriformis muscle resulting strangulated and irritated of sciatic nerve. Piriformis syndrome is mostly seen in the fourth to fifth decade, with female predominance in a ratio of 6 to 1. Prevalence of piriformis syndrome is estimated between 12.2 and 27%. Etiology of this syndrome is divided into primary and secondary causes. Primary piriformis syndrome is related to the anatomical location of piriformis muscle and sciatic nerve with occurrence in 15% of cases whereas secondary piriformis syndrome is caused by repetitive precipitating factors, including microtrauma, macrotrauma, and local ischemia. History of trauma in the pelvic and gluteus regions is a predisposing factor that is often obtained as a trigger for piriformis syndrome. Some individuals who have a high risk of secondary piriformis syndrome are skiers, tennis players, and long distance bicycle athletes.

Piriformis syndrome patients complain of pain in the gluteus area which generally radiates to the lower limbs that may be accompanied by paresthesia, hyperesthesia, and muscle weakness. However, the associated symptoms often indicate a delay in the diagnosis of piriformis syndrome. Delayed diagnosis of piriformis syndrome might lead to various pathologic conditions of sciatic nerve, chronic somatic dysfunction, and compensatory pain. In serious cases, misdiagnosis lead to unnecessary surgery in prolapsed intervertebral disc. The biggest problem of clinical diagnosis of piriformis syndrome is the absence of a specific and consistent test in diagnosing piriformis syndrome. Confirmation of the diagnosis is also as a treatment of piriformis syndrome is imaging guided block injections done by a skilled clinician. Therefore, discovering the characteristics and predisposing factors is expected to aid the primary clinician in sharpening the diagnosis of piriformis syndrome.

K. Mohan Iyer (✉)
Bangalore, Karnataka 560003, India
e-mail: kmiyer28@hotmail.com

K. M. Iyer (ed.), *Piriformis Syndrome*,
https://doi.org/10.1007/978-3-031-40736-9_3

1. Anatomical variation: Location of the sciatic nerve in relationship to the piriformis muscle may lead to piriformis syndrome for example in some cases it pierces the muscle of piriformis which leads to compression.
2. Direct trauma or injury to the buttock leads to a heamatoma causing compression of the sciatic nerve.
3. Excessive siting results in compression which may be known as wallet sciatica or fat wallet syndrome.This is noticed as a discomfort on prolonged sitting.
4. Repitative movements like long distance walking,running or cycling can result in hypertrophy of the piriformis leading to sciatic nerve irritation or enlargent causing compression.

Aetiology of PS

K. Mohan Iyer

1. Anatomic anomalies such as bipartite piriformis muscle or the sciatic nerve course/branching variations with respect to the piriformis muscle as seen in >80% of the population, the sciatic nerve courses deep to and exits inferiorly to the piriformis muscle belly/tendon.

   It is also known to occur in early (proximal) divisions of the sciatic nerve into its tibial and common peroneal components can predispose patients to piriformis syndrome, with these branches passing through and below the piriformis muscle or above and below the muscle.
2. Buttock Pain: Piriformis syndrome causes radiating pain originating in the buttock which may radiate down the leg. The sciatic nerve becomes impinged by the Piriformis muscle, deep in the buttocks resulting in (1) Buttock pain which may (2) may radiate down the back of the thigh and may extend into the calf muscles.
3. Piriformis syndrome is not very common as it causes only about 0.3% to 6% of lower back pain. It may be a painful musculoskeletal condition which may be caused by stretched Piriformis muscle, leading to inflammation of soft tissue, muscle spasms, or both, resulting in nerve compression.
4. Myofascial trigger points may be single like medial piriformis trigger point lies along the piriformis line about an inch outside the edge of the sacrum which is a large, triangular bone at the base of the spine or double which refer pain and tenderness to the sacroiliac joint, gluteal, and hip regions.
5. Predisposing anatomic variants namely 6 types such as:

   Type A: typical pattern with the SN passing below the PM, undivided
   Type B: the CPN exits through the PM and TN exits below the PM
   Type C: the CPN exits above the PM and TN and below the PM
   Type D: the SN exits through the PM, as a single trunk

K. Mohan Iyer (✉)
Bangalore, Karnataka 560003, India
e-mail: kmiyer28@hotmail.com

K. M. Iyer (ed.), *Piriformis Syndrome*,
https://doi.org/10.1007/978-3-031-40736-9_4

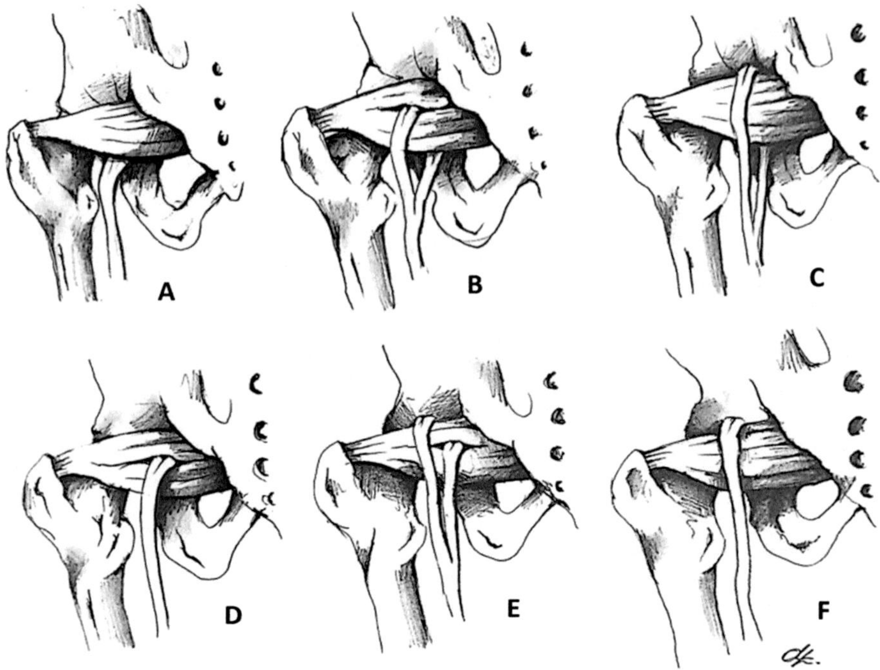

Fig. 1 The Beaton and Anson classification system (1937). [Courtesy: Figure reproduced with the kind permission of Dr. Frideriki Poutoglidou, M.D., M.Sc.]

Type E: the CPN exits above the PM and TN through the PM, and
Type F: the SN passes undivided above the PM as seen in the Fig. 1.

6. Secondary to laminectomy leading to Acute Sciatic Neuritis.
7. Bursitis of the Piriformis muscle: It can also occur in the buttocks when it is called ischial bursitis wic can be symptomatic and seen as pain when sitting or lying down or pain at the back of the thigh or swelling with redness in the affected area.
8. Degenerative disc disease: This happens with due to age and may cause pain in the buttocks and thighs at times with numbness and tingling in the legs which increases on sitting, lifting or bending.
9. Pilonidal cyst which may be found in the cleft between a person's buttocks and differs in containing tiny bits of hair and skin.
10. Perianal abscess which may be infected and filled with pus.
11. Sacroiliac joint dysfunction resulting in pain in the lower back, buttocks, and upper legs.
12. Arthritis of the hips giving rise to raditing pain in te lower back, hips and thighs.
13. Vascular disease may experience pain radiating in the buttocks due to blockage of blood vessels.

Specific Tests for the Piriformis Syndrome

K. Mohan Iyer

The most popular tests are the FAIR test, Beatty maneuver, Freiberg test and the Pace test.

1. FAIR test: Piriformis syndrome is identified by hip flexion, adduction, and internal rotation. It is a nerve-conduction velocity and is expressed as a difference score (nerve-conduction velocity in an aggravating posture minus nerve-conduction velocity in a neutral posture). The larger the FAIR test score, the more likely a patient will have Piriformis syndrome (Fig. 1).
2. Beatty maneuver: When the examiner exerts a slight resistance to the abduction with a hand placed on the knee of the patient. The maneuver is positive when the pain is reported in the buttock and [not in the lumbar spine], while the patient actively abducts the leg.

    Beatty maneuver: Fig. 2 reproduced with the kind permission of Mariana Barzu [PhD, Lecturer West University of Timișoara, Faculty of Physical Education and Sports]; Courtesy: Diagnostic Methods in Piriformis Syndrome which appeared in Timișoara Physical Education and Rehabilitation Journal Volume 6 ◆ Issue 11 ◆ 2013.

1 Modified Beatty Maneuver

Figure 3 reproduced with the kind permission of Mariana Barzu [PhD, Lecturer West University of Timișoara, Faculty of Physical Education and Sports]; Courtesy: Diagnostic Methods in Piriformis Syndrome which appeared in Timișoara Physical Education and Rehabilitation Journal Volume 6 ◆ Issue 11 ◆ 2013.

K. Mohan Iyer (✉)
Bangalore, Karnataka 560003, India
e-mail: kmiyer28@hotmail.com

K. M. Iyer (ed.), *Piriformis Syndrome*,
https://doi.org/10.1007/978-3-031-40736-9_5

Fig. 1 FAIR Test: Figure reproduced with the kind permission of Mariana Barzu [PhD, Lecturer West University of Timișoara, Faculty of Physical Education and Sports]; Courtesy: Diagnostic Methods in Piriformis Syndrome which appeared in Timișoara Physical Education and Rehabilitation Journal Volume 6 ◆ Issue 11 ◆ 2013

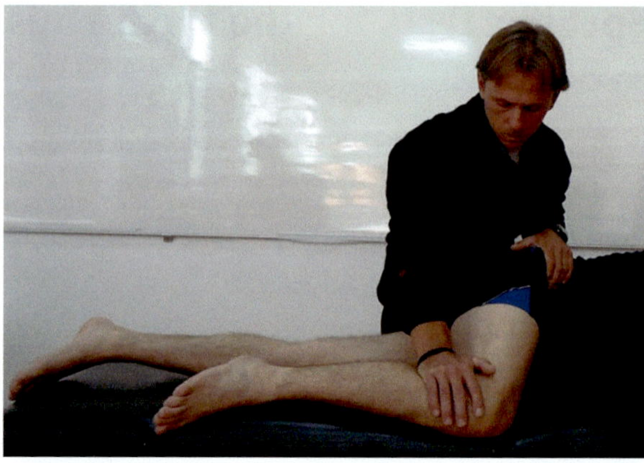

Fig. 2 Beatty maneuver

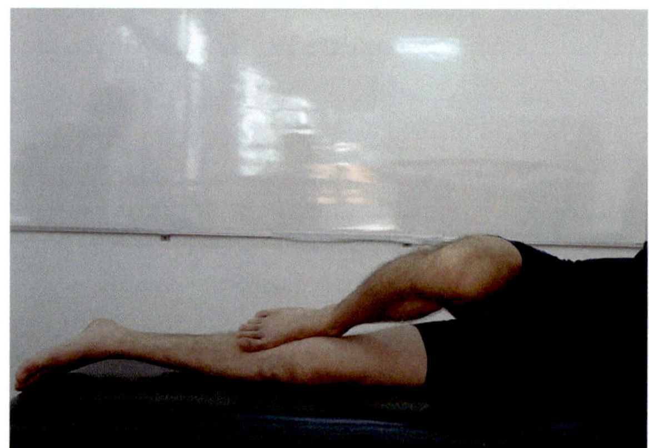

Fig. 3 Modified Beatty maneuver

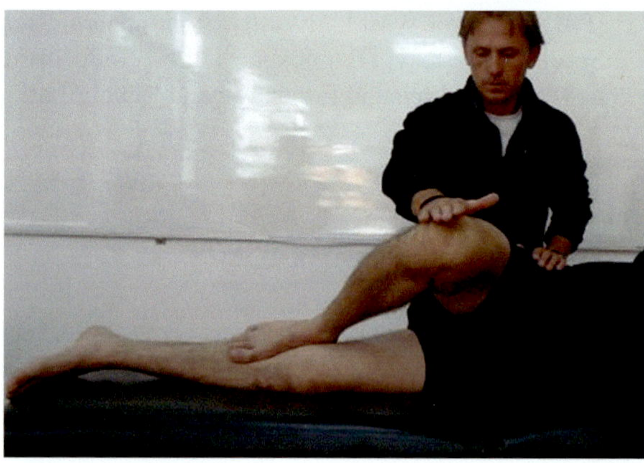

Fig. 4 Figure reproduced with the kind permission of Mariana Barzu [PhD, Lecturer West University of Timișoara, Faculty of Physical Education and Sports]; Courtesy: Diagnostic Methods in Piriformis Syndrome which appeared in Timișoara Physical Education and Rehabilitation Journal Volume 6 ◆ Issue 11 ◆ 2013

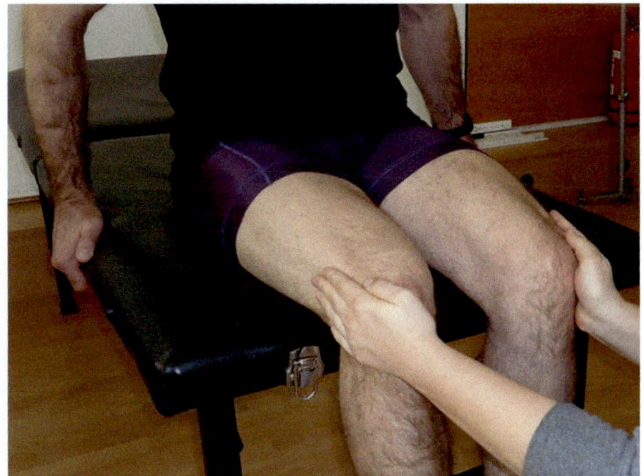

3. Freiberg's maneuver: Freiberg's test produces pain by passively internal rotation of the extended hip, when the patient is in supine. The purpose of this test is on the one hand stretching of the irritated piriformis muscle and also provoking sciatic nerve compression.

4. Pace maneuver: In this test which is a simple diagnostic maneuver, pain in elicited by having the patient abduct the legs in the seated position, which causes a contraction of the piriformis muscle. This maneuver performed by the patient lying with the painful side up, the painful leg flexed, and the knee resting on the table. Buttock pain is produced when the patient lifts and holds the knee several inches off the table. This mainly results in contraction of the piriformis muscle. This test was documented by Pace in 1976 (Fig. 4).

   The modified Pace test: The patient is positioned in a supine relaxed position with the legs hanging off the table at the knees, will be asked to push his legs medially against the resistance provided by the examiner's hands. This movement will produce pain in the deep buttock in a piriformis syndrome (Fig. 5).

5. Heel contralateral knee maneuver (HCLK): This is performed with the patient supine when he is asked to externally rotate the hip to be tested and place the heel on the contralateral knee while the examiner then flexes the patient's contralateral hip and the patient has gluteal pain with or without parasthesia over the posterior aspect of the lower limb and hoding it further for a minute in order to elicit symptoms.

6. Straight leg raise test: With the patient in a supine relaxed position, both legs extended on the couch, the examiner raises the leg on the side to be examined by supporting it with one hand at the ankle, until pain is reported. Usually if pain appears at an angle of 0° 35° of straight leg flexion, the pain is elicited by a piriformis syndrome or/and a sacro iliac joint restriction (Fig. 6).

7. Bonnet test: With the patient in a passive supine position. The examiner realizes a straight leg raise on the affected side, with the hip adducted and realizes an

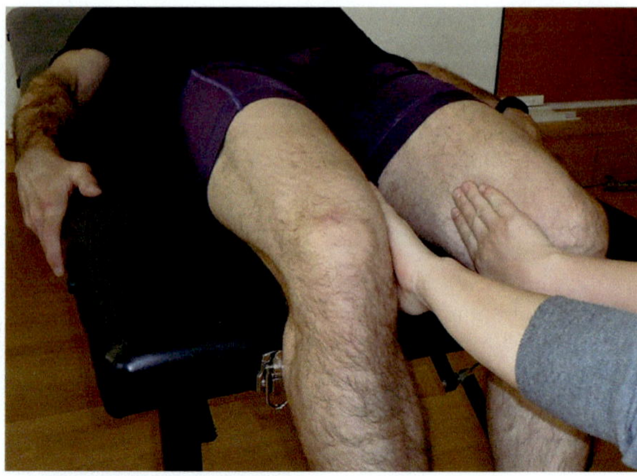

Fig. 5 Figure reproduced with the kind permission of Mariana Barzu [PhD, Lecturer West University of Timișoara, Faculty of Physical Education and Sports]; Courtesy: Diagnostic Methods in Piriformis Syndrome which appeared in Timișoara Physical Education and Rehabilitation Journal Volume 6 ♦ Issue 11 ♦ 2013

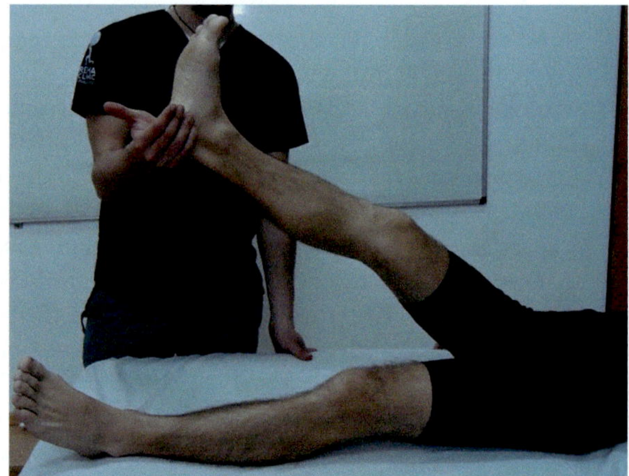

Fig. 6 Figure reproduced with the kind permission of Mariana Barzu [PhD, Lecturer West University of Timișoara, Faculty of Physical Education and Sports]; Courtesy: Diagnostic Methods in Piriformis Syndrome which appeared in Timișoara Physical Education and Rehabilitation Journal Volume 6 ♦ Issue 11 ♦ 2013

     internal rotation of the thigh by supporting with one hand the calf and with the other hand stabilizing the knee. The test will be positive if pain or paresthesia are reported, being specific for sciatica and piriformis syndrome (Fig. 7).

8. Mirkin test: The examiner exerts a pressure into the buttock where the sciatic nerve crosses the piriformis muscle and asks the patient to bend slowly to the floor. If the movement elicits a deep buttock pain the test is positive (Fig. 8).

9. The Piriformis muscle stretch: With the patient in a side lying position, with the affected side up and the hip flexed at 90 degrees, the examiner with one hand on the knee adducts the flexed hip while retracting the ilium with the other hand. This movement will elicit an almost isolated stretch of the piriformis muscle (Fig. 9).

10. Bragard test: It is used to determine whether the source of lower back pain is nervous or muscular. The patient is in a passive supine position. The examiner, supporting with one hand the ankle, raises the leg of the patient in a straight

Fig. 7 Figure reproduced
with the kind permission of
Mariana Barzu [PhD,
Lecturer West University of
Timișoara, Faculty of
Physical Education and
Sports]; Courtesy:
Diagnostic Methods in
Piriformis Syndrome which
appeared in Timișoara
Physical Education and
Rehabilitation Journal
Volume 6 ◆ Issue 11 ◆ 2013

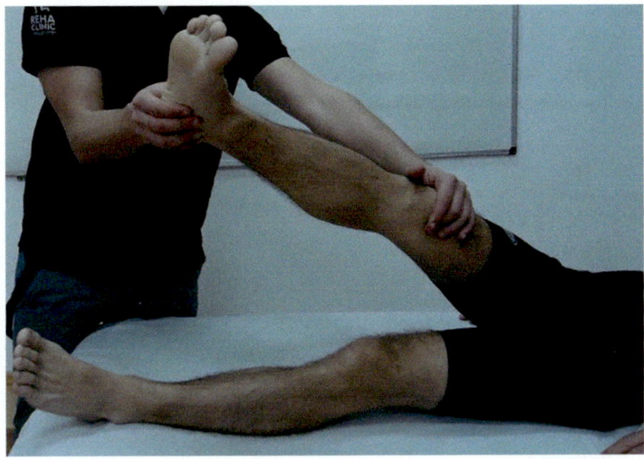

Fig. 8 Figure reproduced
with the kind permission of
Mariana Barzu [PhD,
Lecturer West University of
Timișoara, Faculty of
Physical Education and
Sports]; Courtesy:
Diagnostic Methods in
Piriformis Syndrome which
appeared in Timișoara
Physical Education and
Rehabilitation Journal
Volume 6 ◆ Issue 11 ◆ 2013

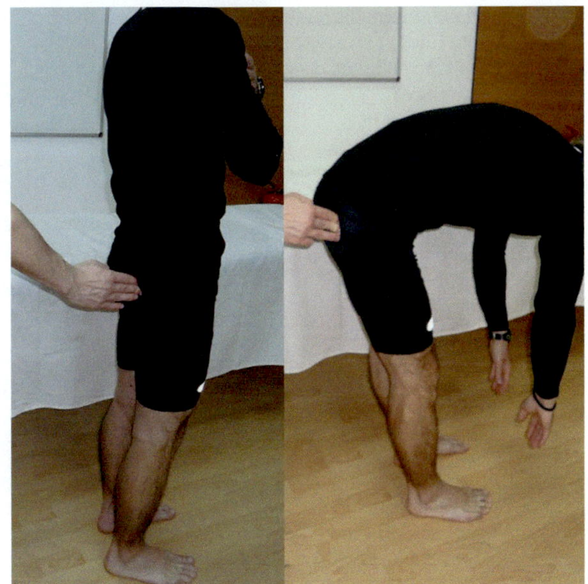

position to the point of pain and then lowers it 5° and with the other hand
dorsiflexes the ankle. If the pain increses during dorsiflexion the pain is likely
of nervous origin. If the pain during dorsiflexion presents no exchange in the
intensity then the source is presumed muscular. Usually, if pain appears at
an angle of 0° 35° of straight leg flexion, the pain is elicited by a piriformis
syndrome or/and a sacro iliac joint restriction (Fig. 10).

Fig. 9 Figure reproduced
with the kind permission of
Mariana Barzu [PhD,
Lecturer West University of
Timișoara, Faculty of
Physical Education and
Sports];Courtesy: Diagnostic
Methods in Piriformis
Syndrome which appeared in
Timișoara Physical
Education and
Rehabilitation Journal
Volume 6 ◆ Issue 11 ◆ 2013

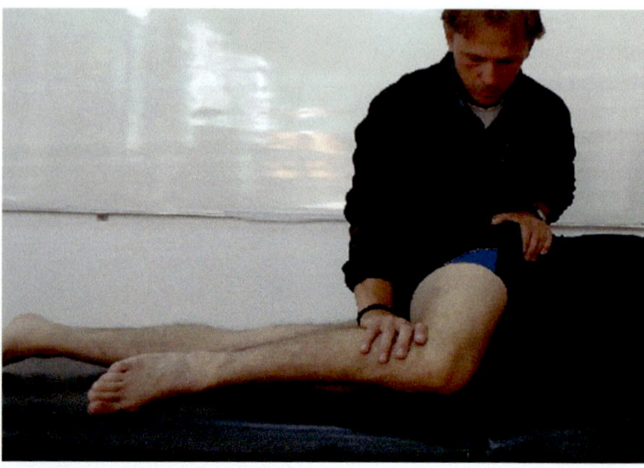

Fig. 10 Figure reproduced
with the kind permission of
Mariana Barzu [PhD,
Lecturer West University of
Timișoara, Faculty of
Physical Education and
Sports]; Courtesy:
Diagnostic Methods in
Piriformis Syndrome which
appeared in Timișoara
Physical Education and
Rehabilitation Journal
Volume 6 ◆ Issue 11 ◆ 2013

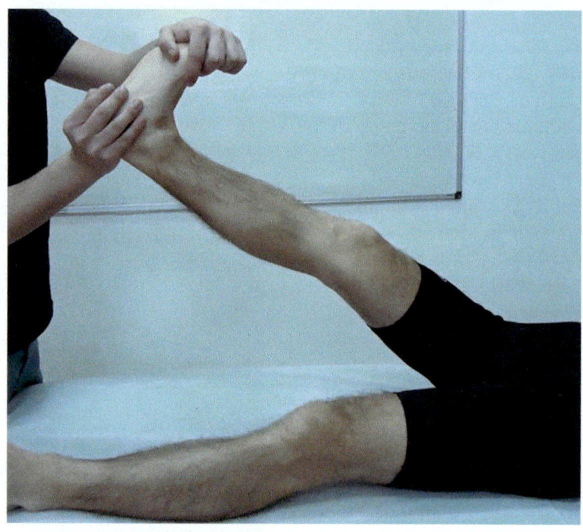

Pathophysiology

K. Mohan Iyer

There are 2 components that is seen in its clinical presentation namely Somatic and Neuropathic.

The somatic component is comprised of a few muscles such as the small external rotators of the hip especially obturator interned which is partly intrapelvic and partly a hip muscle. The neuropathic component refers to the irritation or compression of the sciatic nerve along with neighbouring nerves and vessels which may give rise to pain.

A number of etiological factors that may account for the presence of PS such as previous gluteal trauma which is the most common cause resulting in sciatica-like pain.

Certain anatomic variants, course variations of the sciatic nerve and double piriformis, posterior cutaneous femoral nerve, superior gluteal nerve and the inferior gluteal nerve.

K. Mohan Iyer (✉)
Bangalore, Karnataka 560003, India
e-mail: kmiyer28@hotmail.com

Differential Diagnosis

K. Mohan Iyer

There are numerous conditions with identical symptoms and presentation as follows:

1. Lumbar Disc herniation: This is the commonest in the age group between 35 and 50 which pushes the spinal cord against the nearby spinal root which results in shooting pain in the buttocks and down the leg.
2. Sacroiliac joint dysfunction: Primary involvement of the sacroiliac joint may be seen in cases of instability of hypermobility resulting in lower back pain with radiation to the groin. Even rigidity may result in muscle spasm and pain which may radiate down the back of the leg just like sciatica,
3. Sciatic Neuropathy: This is a painful condition which may be neoplastic, compressive, hereditary, traumatic or iatrogenic.
4. Obturator Internus Muscle: Obturator Internus muscle may result in compression of the sciatic nerve at the infrapiriform foramen due to entrapment between the piriformis and obturator internus muscles.
5. Co-Morbidities like herniated disc, failed back syndrome, complex regional pain syndrome. Spinal stenosis, facet syndrome and sacroiliac syndrome.
6. Trochanteric birsitiis.
7. Ischiofemoral impingement.
8. Unrecognised pelvic fracture.
9. Iliac vien thrombosis.
10. Coccydynia.
11. Post laminectomy syndrome.
12. Posterior facet syndrome.
13. Lumbar Osteochondromatosis.
14. Undiagnosed renal stones.
15. Ischeal tunnel syndrome.

K. Mohan Iyer (✉)
Bangalore, Karnataka 560003, India
e-mail: kmiyer28@hotmail.com

16. Entrapment of the pudendal nerve: The pudendal nerve runs from the back of the pelvis to near the base of your penis or vagina. It sends messages from genitals, anus and controls the sphincter muscles. Pudendal neuralgia is a condition that causes pain, discomfort, or numbness in your pelvis or genitals when a major nerve in the lower body is damaged or irritated. Muscle relaxants and anti-epileptic medicines which give some relief.
17. Pseudaducular S1 syndrome.
18. Deep gluteal syndrome (DGS) is a disease entity that is characterized by pain or dysesthesia in the buttock area, hip, or posterior thigh and/or radicular pain due to a nondiscogenic sciatic nerve entrapment in the subgluteal space.

Imaging

Ankita Ahuja, Gaurav Kant Sharma, Karthikeyan P. Iyengar, and Rajesh Botchu

There is a spectrum of causes for hip pain. One of the uncommon causes for deep hip pain is piriformis syndrome. In this article we discuss the anatomy, pathology and management of piriformis syndrome.

Piriformis syndrome is a rare cause of buttock and hip pain and accounts for 0.3–6% of all back and sciatic pain cases (Hicks et al. n.d.). It is a neuropathic condition and is caused by entrapment of sciatic nerve by the pyriformis muscle. Although it remains a controversial syndrome and a diagnosis of exclusion. It is more common in females as compared to the males, with a ratio of approximately 6:1 (Hicks et al. n.d.; Lee et al. 2004). MRI (Magnetic Resonance Imaging) plays an important role in diagnosis of pyriformis syndrome with ultrasound playing a role in management.

1 Radiological Anatomy

Piriformis muscle is a small pyramidal shaped muscle, arises from the anterior surface of the sacrum at S2 to S4 levels, anterior capsule of the sacroiliac joint and anterior sacro-iliac ligament. It traverses laterally across the greater sciatic foramen to insert onto the apex of greater trochanter as tendon (Khan and Nelson 2018; Standring 2021). The muscle contributes to external rotation of the hip joint and abduction of

A. Ahuja
Innovision Imaging, Mumbai, India

G. K. Sharma
Jaipur Institute of Pain & Sports Injuries (JIPSI), Jaipur, India

K. P. Iyengar
Southport and Ormskirk Hospital NHS Trust, Southport, UK

R. Botchu (✉)
Department of Musculoskeletal Radiology, Royal Orthopedic Hospital, Birmingham, UK
e-mail: drbrajesh@yahoo.com

the thigh in flexed position (Lewis et al. 2016) (Figs. 1 and 2). It is innervated by L5, S1 and S2.

It divides the greater sciatic foramen into the suprapiriform and infrapiriform compartments. The sciatic nerve, inferior gluteal nerves and vessels, posterior femoral cutaneous nerve and nerve to quadratus femoris traverse through the infrapiriform compartment and superior gluteal nerve and vessels traversing through the suprapiriform compartment (Khan and Nelson 2018).

Sciatic nerve is the largest nerve carrying ventral rami of L4-S3 spinal nerves. It descends along the inferior border of pyriformis muscle into the posterior aspect of

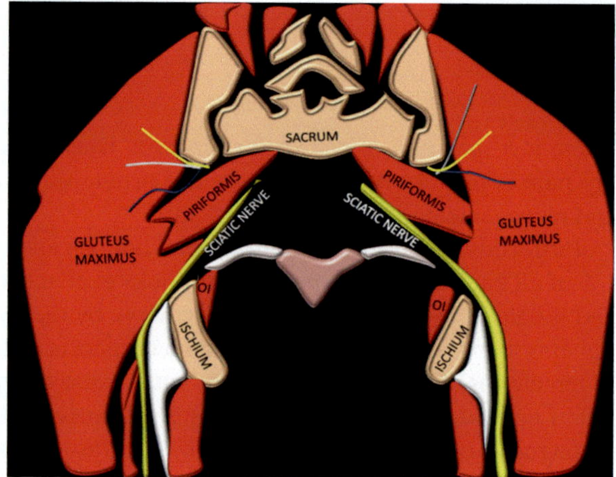

Fig. 1 Schematic coronal of pelvis showing piriformis and sciatic nerve. OI—obturator internus

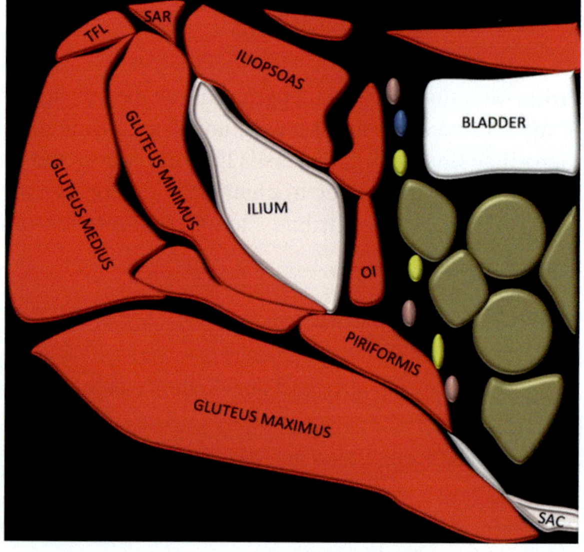

Fig. 2 Axial schematic of right hip showing piriformis. OI—obturator internus, TFL (tensor fascia lata, SAR—sartorius, SAC—sacrum

the thigh and divides into the tibial and common peroneal components in the popliteal fossa (Drake et al. 2005).

2   Anatomical Variations

In majority of population (90%), the sciatic nerve courses the greater sciatic foramen just inferior to the piriformis muscle. However, variations are seen and Beaton performed an anatomic investigation of 216 specimens to determine the possible anatomic variations in relation of the sciatic nerve to the piriformis muscle (Beaton and Anson 1938). In the study, 7.1% population demonstrated that the anterior and posterior divisions of the nerve pass through the divided piriformis muscle, in 2.1% the nerve passed above and below an undivided muscle and in 0.8% an undivided nerve passes through the 2 heads of divided pyriform muscle.

Beaton and Anson classified the anatomical relationship between the sciatic nerve and the piriformis muscle as described in (Table 1) (Lewis et al. 2016; Jha and Baral 2020; Poutoglidou et al. 2020; Natsis et al. 2014) (Fig. 3).

Table 1   Beaton and Anson classification

Types	Beaton and Anson classification
Type A	Undivided nerve below undivided muscle
Type B	Divisions of nerve between and below undivided muscle
Type C	Divisions above and below undivided muscle
Type D	Undivided nerve between heads
Type E	Divisions between and above heads
Type F	Undivided nerve above undivided muscle

Fig. 3   Schematic of the Beaton and Anson classification

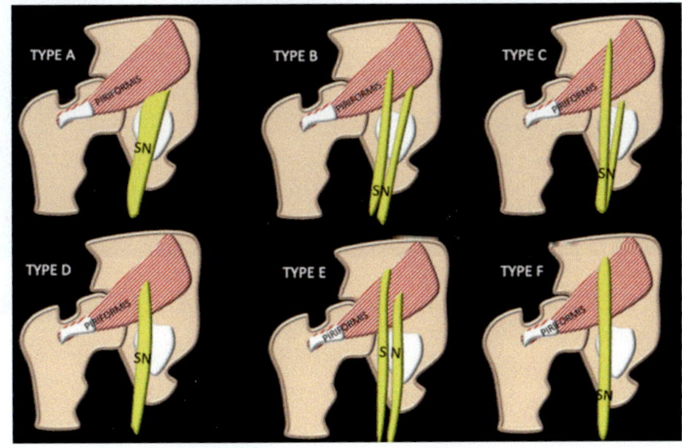

3   Etiology

Piriformis syndrome remains a controversial entity and is often considered to be a diagnosis of exclusion. There are various aetiologies proposed for pyriformis syndrome, post exclusion of the lumbar spinal pathologies. Papadopoulos suggested classification of piriformis syndrome etiologies into primary and secondary (Hicks et al. n.d.) (Table 2). Primary piriformis syndrome is related to the abnormality of the pyriformis muscle and secondary pyriformis syndrome include all other aetiologies excluding the lumbar spinal pathologies (Papadopoulos et al. 1990). The common causes of primary piriformis syndrome include trauma to the hip or buttock area, muscle hypertrophy (often seen in athletes), sitting for prolonged periods and anatomical variations (Fig. 4).

The common secondary causes include neoplastic aetiologies or inferior gluteal artery pseudoaneurysm (Hicks et al. n.d.) (Figs. 5 and 6) (Table 2).

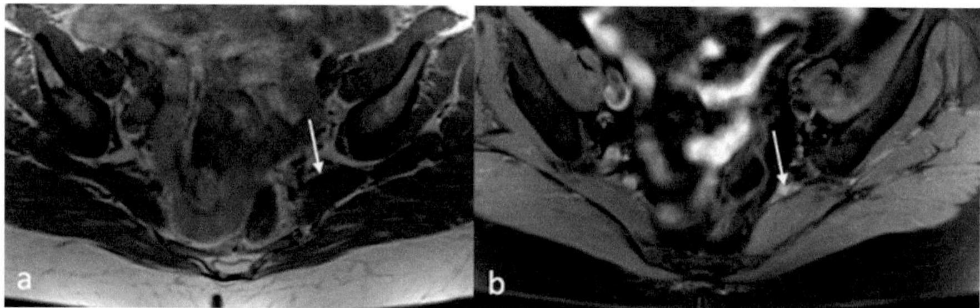

Fig. 4   Axial T1 (a) and PDFS (proton density fat suppressed) showing bulky left piriformis (arrow)

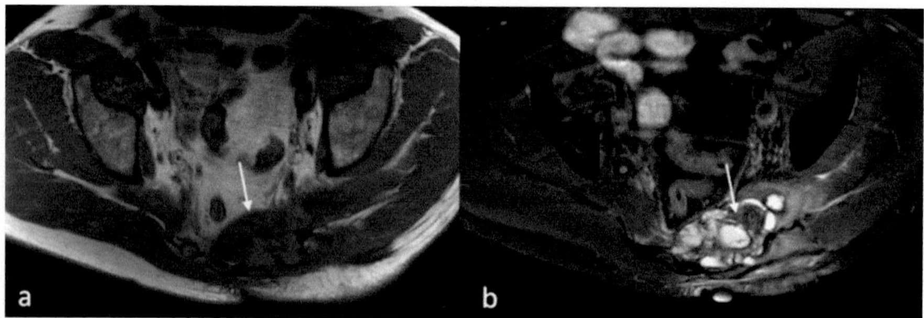

Fig. 5   Axial T1 (a) and STIR (b) showing tumour involving the left piriformis (arrow)

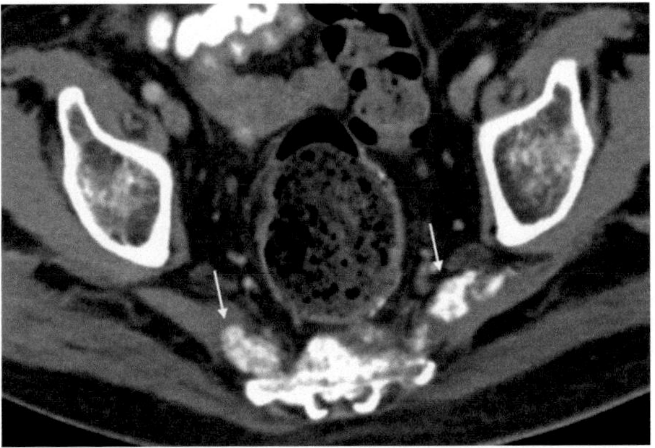

Fig. 6 Axial CT showing calcification within both piriformis

Table 2 Etiologies of pyriformis syndrome

1. Primary piriformis syndrome	Trauma to hip or buttock
	Muscle hypertrophy
	Sitting for prolonged periods
	Anatomical variants
2. Secondary piriformis syndrome	Neoplastic etiologies
	Aneurysm or pseudoaneurysm

4 Imaging Modalities in Piriformis Syndrome

Piriformis syndrome is usually a diagnosis of exclusion and is primarily based on clinical findings (Vassalou et al. 2017). However, imaging modalities play a critical component in assisting the diagnosis. CT (Computed Tomography) and MRI are the primary modalities, of which, MRI is preferred modality due to its better soft tissue resolution. It depicts the piriformis muscle, sciatic nerve and helps to exclude other possible causes for sciatic nerve entrapment. Although, there is no gold standard modality for the diagnosis (Vassalou et al. 2017). High resolution ultrasonography is also being widely applied in view of being more accessible and cost effective.

5 MRI

MRI of the spine is performed first to exclude an intraspinal aetiology which is a common cause of pain. This is followed by MRI of the pelvis in a case of suspicion for piriformis syndrome (Lee et al. 2004).

Considering the various aetiologies, the imaging findings are variable. The most common imaging feature is asymmetry of the piriformis muscle, most commonly hypertrophy, however, in certain cases atrophy can also be seen on the affected site (Jankiewicz et al. 1991; Hughes et al. 1992). Increased T2 signal within the muscle on the ipsilateral side can also be seen.

Sciatic nerve may or may not reveal signal hyperintensity at the level of sciatic notch. MR neurography (MRN) can also be used to evaluate the sciatic nerve. Various studies have shown high specificity and sensitivity (93 and 64%) of piriformis muscle enlargement and sciatic nerve hyperintensity at the level of sciatic notch for diagnosing pyriformis syndrome (Vassalou et al. 2017).

MRI also helps in identifying the variant anatomy and relation of the piriformis muscle with sciatic nerve as described by Beaton and Anson classification which might be the cause of symptoms. Thus, helping in management and pre-operative planning.

Other causes like hematoma or abscess within the piriformis muscle can also be detected on MRI.

Apart from diagnosing primary piriformis syndrome, MRI also helps in diagnosing secondary pyriformis syndrome. It identifies any lesion/neoplastic etiology at the level of greater sciatic notch, responsible for sciatic nerve irritation and piriformis syndrome.

6 Ultrasound

High resolution ultrasonography is being used more widely for evaluation of piriformis muscle to diagnose piriformis syndrome. Ultrasound reveals enlarged and increased echogenicity of the muscle on the symptomatic side as compared to the asymptomatic side. Ultrasound can be used to measure pyriformis muscle thickness which is increased on the symptomatic side (Zhang et al. 2019). A study by YMT Siahaan et al. proposed a cut-off of 0.9950 cm for piriformis muscle thickness for diagnosing piriformis syndrome (Siahaan et al. 2021). Cross sectional area and sciatic nerve diameter are few other measurements which can be obtained on ultrasound (Figs. 7 and 8).

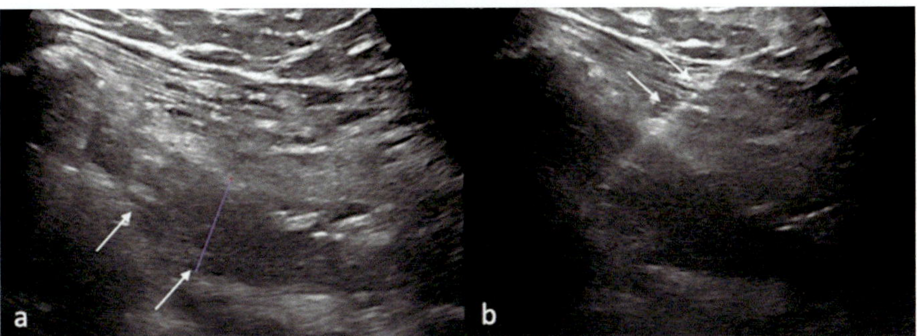

Fig. 7 Ultrasound images showing bulky piriformis which is moderately hypoechoic (arrow) (a) and ultrasound guided injection with needle tip within the piriformis (b) (arrow)

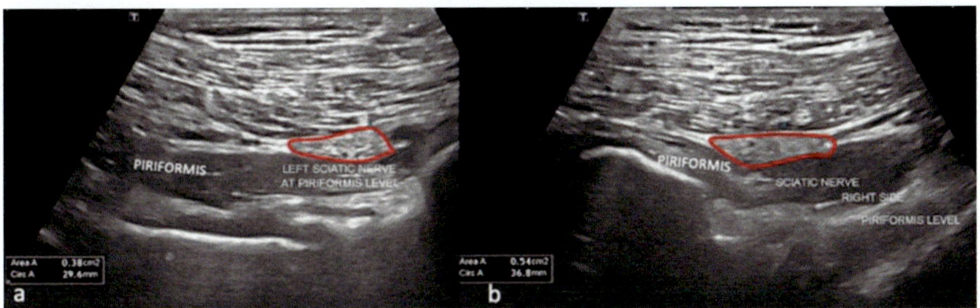

Fig. 8 Ultrasound image showing increased cross-sectional area of sciatic nerve measuring 54 mm^2 on right side (b) as compared to the normal side sciatic nerve measuring 38 mm^2 (a)

7 Other Modalities

Bone scan is rarely performed but can demonstrate increased radiotracer uptake in the piriformis muscle on the affected site (Karl 1985). Electromyography (EMG) may also aid in establishing the diagnosis in patients with non-specific findings on MRI or ultrasound.

Each modality has its pros and cons. MRI with its excellent soft tissue resolution is most commonly used, although it is expensive, relatively less accessible and has longer imaging time. CT has short imaging time but relatively less soft tissue resolution compared to the MRI. Ultrasound is simple, easily accessible and cost-effective technique but is operator dependent. EMG has low specificity and poor repeatability (Hicks et al. n.d.).

8 Management

Piriformis syndrome is usually treated conservatively. The conservative approach includes pharmacologic therapy including non-steroidal anti-inflammatory drugs (NSAIDs) and muscle relaxants, physiotherapy and lifestyle modifications (Lee et al. 2004; Benzon et al. 2003).

Steroid (Hicks et al. n.d.; Smith et al. 2006) and botulinum toxin (Lang 2004) injections are also commonly used in the treatment of piriformis syndrome. The injection is performed into the pyriformis muscle. Fluoroscopy with or without muscle electromyography and ultrasonography are used to perform the injections (Benzon et al. 2003).

8.1 Ultrasound Guided Injections

Ultrasound-guided injections are real time with minimal morbidity to the patient. It also provides an opportunity for a real-time assessment of the patient's response to the injection (Benzon et al. 2003; Smith et al. 2006; Bardowski and Byrd 2019).

8.2 Technique

The patient is placed in the prone position with the lower extremities in neutral rotation and feet just off the edge of the examination table. Typically, a low-frequency curvilinear transducer is used because of the depth of the piriformis muscle. A lower-frequency linear probe can potentially be used for patients with a small body habitus. Prior to the injection, muscle and sciatic nerve are identified (Fig. 7). A Doppler scan is done to locate vessels. Standard sterile precautions are used and cleaning, draping of the area is performed. The medications are injected under direct visualization. The needle is withdrawn, and a small bandage is applied.

8.3 Fluoroscopy Guided Injection

In fluoroscopy guided injection, patient is place prone and an AP (Anteroposterior) radiograph is performed to demonstrate the inferior most part of the sacroiliac joint in the middle. The target decided is 1 cm inferior and 1 cm lateral to the SI joint. Standard sterile precautions are used. Local anaesthesia is administered in the skin and deep soft tissues. The needle is then advanced to the target site. A change in resistance may be noticed on entering the muscle. Contrast is injected and demonstrates a diagonal spread. Following this, the medications are injected.

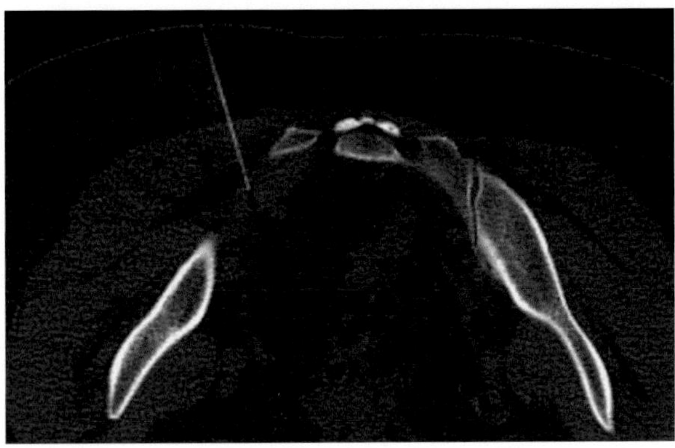

Fig. 9 Axial CT images showing needle with tip in the piriformis muscle

8.4 CT Guided Injection

CT-guided piriformis injection is also a safe and effective method in the treatment of piriformis syndrome (Akdemir Ozisik et al. n.d.; Masala et al. 2012) (Fig. 9).

References

Akdemir Ozisik P, Toru M, Denk CC, Taskiran OO, Gundogmus B. CT-guided piriformis muscle injection for the treatment of piriformis syndrome.

Bardowski EA, Byrd JT. Piriformis injection: an ultrasound-guided technique. Arthrosc Tech. 2019;8(12):e1457–61.

Beaton LE, Anson BJ. The sciatic nerve and the piriformis muscle: their interrelation a possible cause of coccygodynia. JBJS. 1938;20(3):686–8.

Benzon HT, Katz JA, Benzon HA, Iqbal MS. Piriformis syndrome: anatomic considerations, a new injection technique, and a review of the literature. J Am Soc Anesthesiologists. 2003;98(6):1442–8.

Drake RL, Gray H, Vogl W, Mitchell AW. Gray's anatomy for students. Elsevier Health Sciences TW; 2005.

Hicks BL, Lam JC, Varacallo M. Piriformis syndrome.

Hughes SS, Goldstein MN, Hicks DG, Pellegrini Jr VD. Extrapelvic compression of the sciatic nerve. An unusual cause of pain about the hip: report of five cases. JBJS. 1992;74(10):1553–9.

Jankiewicz JJ, Hennrikus WL, Houkom JA. The appearance of the piriformis muscle syndrome in computed tomography and magnetic resonance imaging: a case report and review of the literature. Clin Orthop Relat Res (1976–2007). 1991;262:205–9.

Jha AK, Baral P. Composite anatomical variations between the sciatic nerve and the piriformis muscle: a Nepalese cadaveric study. Case Rep Neurol Med. 2020;31:2020.

Karl Jr RD, Yedinak MA, Hartshorne MF, Cawthon MA, Bauman JM, Howard WH, Bunker SR. Scintigraphic appearance of the piriformis muscle syndrome. Clin Nucl Med. 1985;10(5):361–3.

Khan D, Nelson A. Piriformis syndrome. In: Essentials of pain medicine. Elsevier; 2018. p. 613–18.

Lang AM. Botulinum toxin type B in piriformis syndrome. Am J Phys Med Rehabil. 2004;83(3):198–202.

Lee EY, Margherita AJ, Gierada DS, Narra VR. MRI of piriformis syndrome. Am J Roentgenol. 2004;183(1):63–4.

Lewis S, Jurak J, Lee C, Lewis R, Gest T. Anatomical variations of the sciatic nerve, in relation to the piriformis muscle. Transl Res Anat. 2016;1(5):15–9.

Masala S, Crusco S, Meschini A, Taglieri A, Calabria E, Simonetti G. Piriformis syndrome: long-term follow-up in patients treated with percutaneous injection of anesthetic and corticosteroid under CT guidance. Cardiovasc Intervent Radiol. 2012;35:375–82.

Natsis K, Totlis T, Konstantinidis GA, Paraskevas G, Piagkou M, Koebke J. Anatomical variations between the sciatic nerve and the piriformis muscle: a contribution to surgical anatomy in piriformis syndrome. Surg Radiol Anat. 2014;36:273–80.

Papadopoulos SM, McGillicuddy JE, Albers JW. Unusual cause of 'piriformis muscle syndrome.' Arch Neurol. 1990;47(10):1144–6.

Poutoglidou F, Piagkou M, Totlis T, Tzika M, Natsis K. Sciatic nerve variants and the piriformis muscle: a systematic review and meta-analysis. Cureus. 2020;12(11).

Siahaan YM, Tiffani P, Tanasia A. Ultrasound-guided measurement of piriformis muscle thickness to diagnose piriformis syndrome. Front Neurol. 2021;7(12): 721966.

Smith J, Hurdle MF, Locketz AJ, Wisniewski SJ. Ultrasound-guided piriformis injection: technique description and verification. Arch Phys Med Rehabil. 2006;87(12):1664–7.

Standring S, editor. Gray's anatomy e-book: the anatomical basis of clinical practice. Elsevier Health Sciences; 2021.

Vassalou EE, Fotiadou A, Ziaka D, Natsiopoulos K, Karantanas AH. Piriformis muscle syndrome: MR imaging findings and treatment outcome in 23 patients. Hellenic J Radiol. 2017;2(4).

Zhang W, Luo F, Sun H, Ding H. Ultrasound appears to be a reliable technique for the diagnosis of piriformis syndrome. Muscle Nerve. 2019;59(4):411–6.

Electro-Diagnostic Studies

Mahmoud Diab Abdelhaleem

Piriformis syndrome (PS) is a myofascial disorder which induces not only deep gluteal pain, but also peripheral neurological symptoms that mimics and could be misdiagnosed as radiculopathy. The peripheral symptoms result from the entrapment of sciatic nerve (SN) by the piriformis muscle (PM) (Nisargandha et al. 2020).

Sciatic neuropathy or sciatica is characterized by persistent sharp pain that travels down to the leg through the sciatic course. It has less favorable outcomes and difficult to diagnose, also it has negative impact on productivity and social life of the affected subject as it consumes health resource and lead to work absentee (Nisargandha et al. 2017; Magladery and McDougal 1950).

Electrodiagnostic testing is useful in the diagnosis process of nerve injuries and lead the ability to specify the location and severity of the injury. It also helpful for determining both recovery period and prognosis potential of the injured nerve. Nerve conduction velocity (NCV) is a critical exam that used to assess the function of the suspected nerve especially the conductivity and the modulation function of that nerves. It can determine the degree of demyelination and axonal loss in the affected nerves (Tsao 2007; Distad and Weiss 2013).

As a classification of severity, NCV could show the degree of demyelination by measuring the of conduction velocity and delay period, The results could indicate nerve compression if this time became longer than normal which reflect decreased velocity or could indicate axonal loss if no conduction velocity recorded from the examined nerves (Mallik and Weir 2005; Najdi et al. 2019).

Najdi and his colleges 2019 nourished the literature with a valuable classification for PS. They depended on latency delay of peroneal nerve (PN) H-reflex for their proposal. They also demonstrated that latency measuring is more reliable than the amplitude changes in PN H-reflex. They classified PS into three grads, High with a

M. D. Abdelhaleem (✉)
Department of Orthopedic Physical Therapy, Faculty of Physical Therapy, Cairo University, 7 Ahmed El Zaiat St., Bein El Sarayat, Giza 12612, Egypt
e-mail: Mahmoud.diab@pt.cu.edu.eg

K. M. Iyer (ed.), *Piriformis Syndrome*,
https://doi.org/10.1007/978-3-031-40736-9_9

delay more than 5 ms, Moderate with a delay between 4 and 5 ms and low with a delay less than 4 ms (Najdi et al. 2019).

Electromyogram (EMG) could help in diagnosing PS, peripheral neuropathy and radiculopathy caused by disc lesions. It could be helpful in diagnosing cases that could not be discovered by MRI as PS or when (NCV) could not rule out different diagnosis. In diagnosis process of radiculopathy caused by compression of nerve roots, EMG could record abnormal signaling of the paraspinal muscles activities as they supplied by corresponding nerve root, although their activities will be recorded normal by EMG in PS as the sciatic nerve been entrapped after emerging from the lumbo-sacral plexus and entered the pelvis (Michel et al. 2013; Fishman et al. 2004; Kulkarni et al. 2015).

As a differentiation tool, EMG studies could help to distinguish between PS and Herniated Inter-Vertebral Disc (HIVD) causing Radiculopathy. EMG for paraspinals muscles is the key stone in this scenario as in radiculopathy cases paraspinal EMG will be abnormal as these muscles innervated by corresponding nerve root, so if theses root got entrapped or compromised the muscles activity will be affected. In the opposite, EMG for paraspinal muscles will be spared in PS as SN is entrapped by PM after it merges from the lumbo-sacral plexus and entering the pelvis and the paraspinal muscles receive their innervation from the nerves which are branching proximal to the site of sciatic entrapment between PM (Najdi et al. 2019; Michel et al. 2013; Kulkarni et al. 2015).

In the same vein NCV readings could be affected by certain maneuvers that used to assess the PS as FAIR maneuver. This maneuver could induce more tension of piriformis muscle and resulted in more compression on sciatic nerve and decrease its conductivity. On the other hand, this maneuver may not affect the sciatic conductivity if the patient has radiculopathy as the excursion of sciatic nerve will be normal (Moon et al. 2015; Fishman et al. 2002).

On the other hand, The EMG could guide the surgeons during operative procedures or local injections to reach the Piriformis muscle to be injected by the ingredient. This was demonstrated by research work performed by Mitchell and his colleges, 2013. During this study they used EMG-guided technique to reach PM to inject it by Botox to compare its effect with conservative and surgical release procedures (Michel et al. 2013).

In the same vein, Fishman, and colleges in 2004 used EMG-guided injection to study the effect of botulinum neurotoxin effect on PS by applying FAIR test. Their study revealed the significancy of EMG during minor surgery and local injections to target deep muscles as PM. This objective method could boost a satisfactory result for both the surgeon and patient (Fishman et al. 2004).

During their research at 2015, Kulkarin and colleges used both NCV and EMG to confirm the diagnosis of PS at 60 years old man who experienced low back with radiation for more than 3 years. They assumed that electro-diagnostics could differentiated PS from radiculopathy and eliminate the need to perform MRI which is expensive and often unaffordable. This case presented with all Freiberg's PS signs (Positive Lasegues sign, positive FAIR test, and tender piriformis muscles). All these symptoms' mimics L5-S1 radiculopathy so the authors performed EMG and NCV to exclude the radiculopathy and rule in the PS hypothesis. EMG-NCV studies showed that H-reflex was absent bilateral and sensory and motor nerve conductions were normal bilateral, so the authors suggested adding FAIR maneuver during EMG study to confirm PS and could help to differentiate between PS and Radiculopathy by HIVD (Kulkarni et al. 2015).

Moon and his college, 2015 examined in their paper a 32-years old female patient who was complaining from bilateral sciatica. She presented with persistent complain of sensory manifestation, ankle dorsiflexor weakness and high steppage gait was obvious. She experienced these symptoms for 6 years in one leg and the other leg symptoms started recently. Scenes hip MRI did not show any evidence of abnormality at both SNs, the authors used EMG to examine this case and it showed abnormal spontaneous activity on left tibialis anterior and gastrocnemius. The MRI of lumbar spine revealed central to right L5-S1 disc bulge and swelling around S1 nerve root. The authors concluded that EMG could help to differentiate between PS and HIVD radiculopathy as in this scenario EMG study did show no abnormal of proximal muscles of L5-S1 myotome (Moon et al. 2015).

Also, Fishman and his colleges in 2002 studied H-reflex on patients diagnosed with PS. They recorded H-reflex from both branches of SN Common Peroneal Nerve (CPN) and Posterior Tibial Nerve (PTN) from anatomical and FAIR test position. All the subjects were presented with 2 or 3 criteria from Frieberg's criteria of PS. The main purpose of this study was to assess the reliability of both H-reflexes. They performed their study on three groups one received surgical treatment and second received injection and third treated with medications. They reported that PS spasm could compress the sciatic nerve and could cause transit delay in NCV of SN during FAIR maneuver. The difference from anatomical and FAIR positions explained by the fact that H-Loops is enlarged as both afferent and efferent limbs of H-reflexes piercing the PS, so any increased tension in PS will directly affect H-reflex and the authors recommended the use stretching and relaxing measures that targets the PS to increase its flexibility and in turn enhance SN functions (Fishman et al. 2002).

In the same way, Najdi et al. (2019) and Jawish et al. (2010) recommended that the use of Common Peroneal Nerve CPN H-reflex is more valid and reliable than posterior tibial nerve PTN in management of patients with PS (Najdi et al. 2019; Michel et al. 2013; Fishman et al. 2004, 2002; Kulkarni et al. 2015; Moon et al. 2015; Jawish et al. 2010).

Najdi and his colleges examined the effect surgical treatment against conservative and injection therapy in three different groups of patients diagnosed with PS. In their study, they observed that CPN H-reflex is much affected by FAIR test position as all conduction studies were delayed, However PTN H-reflex did not show signs of delay or changes in velocity studies (Najdi et al. 2019). These findings are demonstrated that impingement of SN Caused by different compressing elements, predicted that fibers of CPN were more vulnerable because of its posterior location in a direct face with sacrospinous ligament and the PS (Mustafa et al. 2008; Nicolas Roydon Smoll 2010; Natsis et al. 2014).

Therefore, the electrical testing of CPN H-reflex could help in determine the presence of impingement when SN is compressed by PS. In the same manner, Fishman in his study published 1992, Examined PTN H-reflex and they did not observe any significance of the H-reflex delay between patients with PS and control groups during using FAIR maneuver (Fishman and Zybert 1992).

In the seam, Haplin and Ganju (2009) concluded that the tibial division of the sciatic nerve is less frequently involved in PS than CPN, due to the medial location of the PTN into the sciatic notch, and therefore PTN fibers are not initially involved in the impingement syndrome (Haplin and Ganju 2009).

As an objective assessment tool, Abdelhaleem et al. (2022) used NCV during their randomized trial in-which they examined the effect of simultaneous application of position release technique and Maitland mobilization technique on patients with sciatica (Abdelhaleem et al. 2022). The main technique was used to target PS muscles as SN entering the pelvis by passing through it. Piriformis muscles disorders could induce venous congestion around SN which compress SN vasa nervosa which in turn provide less supply to the nerve which resulted in poor nerve functions. Theses pathological changes has been agreed by MRI studies performed by Pacult et al. (2018). The authors concluded that PM position releases technique along with Maitland mobilization technique successfully increased SN conduction abilities in patients with Sciatica (Abdelhaleem et al. 2022).

In conclusion, most of the authors recommend using the NCV-EMG testing to confirm the diagnosis of PS as it was assumed that accurate diagnosis could guide to optimum treatment. Piriformis muscles disorders is the leading cause of PS, these disorders include muscle hypertrophy, hypertonicity, spasm, tightness and inflammation, other causes may include anatomical variations as presence of fibrous band, congested veins, and tight Sacro-spinous ligaments (Kim et al. 2019). The diagnosis of PS could be performed by recording the delay in latency of NCV. The authors prefer the CPN H-reflex as it was proven to be valid and reliable.

References

Abdelhaleem M, Abdallah E, Neamat Allah N, Zaitoon Z, Zahran S, Abdelhay M. Effect of simultaneous application of position releases technique and Maitland mobilization technique on sciatica: a randomized controlled trial. Bulletin of Faculty of Physical Therapy, 2022;27–9.

Distad B, Weiss M. Clinical and electrodiagnostic features of sciatic neuropathy. Phs Med Rehabil Clin N AM. 2013;24:107–20.

Fishman M, Zybert A. Eletrophysiologic evidence of Piriforms syndrome. Arch Phys Med Rehabil. 1992;73(4):359–64.

Fishman M, Dombi W, Michaelsen C, Ringel S, Rozbruch J, Rosner B, Weber C. Piriformis syndrome: diagnosis, Treatment, and outcome—a 10-year study. Arch Med Rehabil. 2002;83:295–301.

Fishman M, Konnoth C, Rozner B. Boutinum neurotoxin type B and physical therapy in the treatment of Piriforms syndrome: a dose-finding Study. AM J Phys Med Rehabil. 2004;83:42–50.

Haplin R, Ganju A. Piriformis syndrome a real pain in the buttock? Neurosurgery. 2009;65:197–202.

Jawish R, Assoum H, Khamis C. Anatomical, clinical and electrical observations in piriformis syndrome. J Orthop Surg Res. 2010;5:3.

Kim H-J, Lee S, Park H, Kim K, Lee Y. Accessory belly of the piriformis muscle as a cause of piriformis syndrome: a case report with magnetic resonance imaging and magnetic resonance neurography imaging findings. iMRI 2019;23:142–7.

Kulkarni R, Borole B, Chaudhary J, Dev S. A case of Piriforms syndrome presenting as radiculopathy. Indian J Pain 2015;29(2).

Magladery JW, McDougal DB. Electrophysiological studies of nerve and reflex activity in normal man, I: identification of certain reflexes in the electromyogram and the conduction velocity of peripheral nerve fibers. Bull Johns Hopkins. 1950;86:265–89.

Mallik A, Weir I. Nerve conduction studies: essentials and pitfalls in practice. J Neurosurg Psychiatry 2005;76.

Michel F, Decavel P, Toussirot E, Tatu L, Aleton E, Monnier G, Garbuio P, Parratte B. Piriformis muscle syndrome: Diagnostic criteria and treatment of a monocentric series of 250 patients. Ann Phys Rehabil Med. 2013;56:371–83.

Moon H, Nam K, Kwon B, Park J, Ryu G, Lee H, Kim C. Leg weakness caused by bilateral Piriforms syndrome: a case report. Ann Rehabil Med, 2015;39(6).

Mustafa G, Pınar A, Cihan I, Süleyman T. Anatomic considerations and the relationship between the piriformis muscle and the sciatic nerve. Surg Radiol Anat. 2008;30:467–74.

Najdi H, Mouarbes D, Abi-akl J, Karnib S, Chamsedine A, Jawish. EMG in Piriforms syndrome diagnosis: reliability of peroneal H-reflex according to results obtained after surgery, Botox injection and medical treatment. J Clin Neurosci. 2019;59:55–61.

Natsis K, Totlis T, Konstantinidis GA, Paraskevas G, Piagkou M, Koebke J. Anatomical variations between the sciatic nerve and the piriformis muscle: a contribution to surgical anatomy in piriformis syndrome. Surg Radiol Anat. 2014;36(3):273–80.

Nisargandha MA, Parwe S, Wankhede S, Shinde P, Phatale S, Deshpande V. Conduction studies on patient with sciatica. Int J Biol Med Res. 2017;8(3).

Nisargandha N, Parwe S, Wankhede S, Deshpande V. Comparison of nerve conduction studies on affected and non-affected side in the patients of sciatica. Int J Basic Appl Physiol. 2020;9(1).

Pacult A, Henderson C, Varma K. Sciatica caused by venous varix compression of the sciatic nerve. World Neurosurg. 2018;117:242–5.

Smoll NR. Variations of the piriformis and sciatic nerve with clinical consequence: a review. Clin Anat. 2010;23:8–17.

Tsao B. The electrodiagnosis of cervical and lumbosacral radiculopathy. Neurol Clin. 2007;25:473–94.

Intrapelvic Causes of Sciatica in Piriformis Syndrome

K. Mohan Iyer

Entrapment neuropathy of the sciatic nerve and pudendal nerve are painful syndromes which are frequently missed by medical personel which are usually identified by laparoscopic surgical interventions for removing the compression lesions which may cause sciatica, as well as pudendal neuralgia. A rare instance caused by aberrant vessels and a variant piriformis muscle bundle may be a cause of sciatic and pudendal nerve entrapment. This was successfully managed by laparoscopic decompression technique for the pudendal and sciatic nerves. The pain pattern which is invariably shooting in nature is along the course of the nerve dermatome leads to its diagnosis (Fig. 1). Endometriosis, fibrotic tissue or vascular entrapment, and piriformis muscle syndrome has also been documented in literature[25].

They reported five etiologies of nerve entrapments identified during surgery in these patients as

1. endometriosis,
2. fibrosis,
3. piriformis entrapment by abnormal muscle fibres originating medial to the sacral foramina,
4. neurovascular conflict, and
5. neoplasm.

With recent advances in laparoscopic surgery, to obtain diagnostic certainty prior to initiating treatment for many intrapelvic nerve pathologies, intrapelvic nerve decompression should be considered for painful syndromes.

K. Mohan Iyer (✉)
Bangalore, India
e-mail: kmiyer28@hotmail.com

K. M. Iyer (ed.), *Piriformis Syndrome*,
https://doi.org/10.1007/978-3-031-40736-9_10

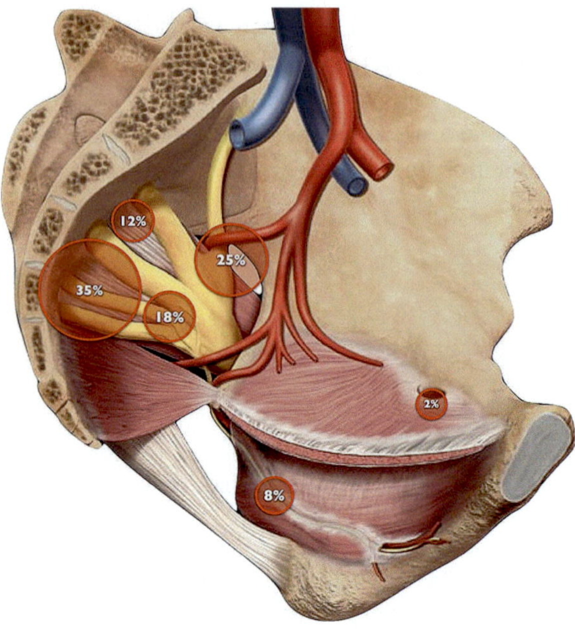

Fig. 1 Distribution of nerve entrapments locations: 35% in proximal S2/S3/S4 nerve roots, 25% in sciati lumbosacral, 18% in proximal pudendal/medial sciatic, 12% in S1/S2 nerve roots, 8% in Alcock's canal level and 2% in obturator nerve entrapment. *Courtesy* Figure reproduced with the kind permission of Dr. Nucelio Lemos, MD, Ph.D.

Presently, intrapelvic entrapments are ill understood and rarely considered as a cause of sciatica or pudendal neuralgia. The main reason being the deep location of retroperitoneal location of the plexus in the pelvis which is best approached by laparoscopy, which provides better lighting, magnification and visualization of this area. The article also described the different locations of entrapments, which is very important for understanding the dermatomes and myotomes implicated in INE [intrapelvic nerve entrapments].

Secondly, lack of awareness of INEs increases risk of patients undergoing ineffective surgeries which cannot address the underlying cause of pain and may cause added harm by excessive consumption of opiods.

Pudendal neuralgia is when a patient has chronic pelvic pain due to damage or irritation to the *pudendal nerve* resulting in stabbing, burning or shooting pain. This pain is mainly occurs during the sitting in buttocks, perineum and genital region.

There are three branches of the pudendal nerve namely a rectal branch, a perineal branch and a clitoral/penile branch and its diagnosis is by

1. Vaginal or Rectal examination
2. Magnetic resonance imaging (MRI)
3. Electromyography [EMG]
4. Nerve blockers.

The most common causes are endometriosis of the sciatic nerve in women, vascular compression and surgical injury to nerves are the most frequent intrapelvic causes of sciatica.

Usually sciatica results when something presses or rubs on the SN or the sacral nerve root (SNR), most causes reported in the literature do not deal with the sciatic nerve itself but rather with pathologies of spinal cord: prolapsed intervertebral disc being the most common cause, followed by spinal stenosis, spondylolisthesis or surgical scarring, trauma and tumors at the level of the lumbar spine. All these causes may affect the sciatic nerve fibers contained in the spinal cord causing direct compression or chemical inflammation, resulting in sciatica. The only cited "intrapelvic cause" for sciatica is piriformis syndrome.

Sacral Plexus Endometriosis or Endometriosis of the Sciatic Nerve and Vascular entrapment of the sacral plexus/sciatic nerve or Surgical damage to the pelvic nerves and Pelvic tumors affecting the pelvic nerves and Sacral tumors/sacroiliac osteochondrosarcoma or Nerve tumors such as Pelvic schwannoma. In some reported cases are also seen in Superior gluteal vein syndrome as an intrapelvic cause of sciatica. A ganglionic cyst can occur in various lesions in the body but seldom around the hip joint.

In an interesting case report with the patient being in the prone position with general anesthesia the gluteus maximus muscle were dissected and retracted. The underlying piriformis muscle and the sciatic nerve were identified after dissection and cutting of the branches of the inferior gluteal artery and vein. An interesting observation made during exploration of the sciatic nerve is that it is not due to the muscle itself, but rather to the piriformis tendon and the sacrotuberous ligament (Fig. 2). In fact on discussion with the author who has experienced a larger number of sciatic nerve entrapment. He recommends complete decompression of the tibial and peroneal divisions of the sciatic nerve with resection of the surrounding pyriformis and its tendinous structure.

In fact he has experienced a huge number of sciatic nerve entrapment so far.

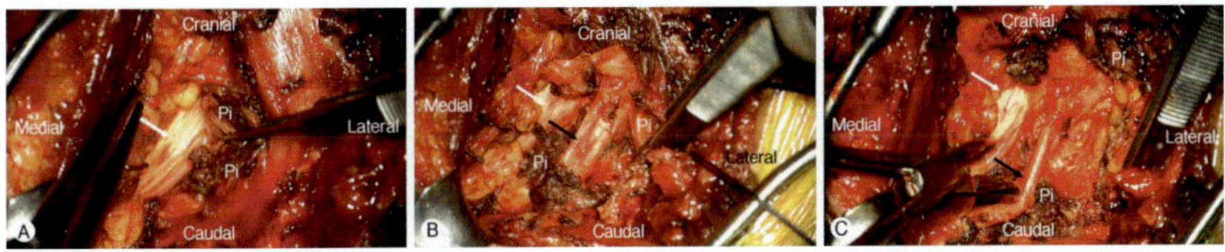

Fig. 2 Courtesy: Figure reproduced with the kind permission of Dr. Byung-chul Son, Department of Neurosurgery, Seoul St. Mary's Hospital, Catholic Neuroscience Institute, College of Medicine, The Catholic University of Korea from his article in The Nerve 2020; 6(2): 114–119

Pyomyositis of the Piriformis Muscle

S. Shanmuga Jayanthan, S. Shanumga Hariharan,
and K. Nadanasadharam

1 Introduction

Piriformis syndrome is a rare cause of sciatica, which results in low backache due to sciatic nerve compression. This syndrome is associated with abnormalities in the piriformis muscle, which cause sciatic nerve entrapment, like anatomical variations, muscle hypertrophy, and inflammation. It can also result from the abnormal course of sciatic nerve itself through normal piriformis muscle. Piriformis syndrome due to pyomyositis of the piriformis muscle is extremely rare and only 23 cases are reported in literature (Shanmuga Jayanthan et al. 2021).

2 Imaging Findings

X ray is often unremarkable. Ultrasound (USG) might show a multi- loculated hypo-echoic collection with peripheral color uptake on Doppler study. However, its utility is limited by the field of view. Hence, cross sectional images are preferred. The abscess is seen as a well defined hypo-dense intra muscular collection on non-contrast CT (Fig. 1).

Contrast enhanced CT (CECT) will show a peripherally enhancing collection with enhancing internal septations, similar to contrast enhanced magnetic resonance image (CE-MRI). MRI is the imaging modality of choice, owing to its high soft tissue contrast resolution. Piriformis abscess is evidenced by a T1 iso-hypo intense and T2 hyper intense intra muscular collection (Figs. 2, and 3).

S. Shanmuga Jayanthan (✉) · S. Shanumga Hariharan · K. Nadanasadharam
Meenakshi Hospital, Tanjore, Tamil Nadu 613005, India
e-mail: jettan.32@gmail.com

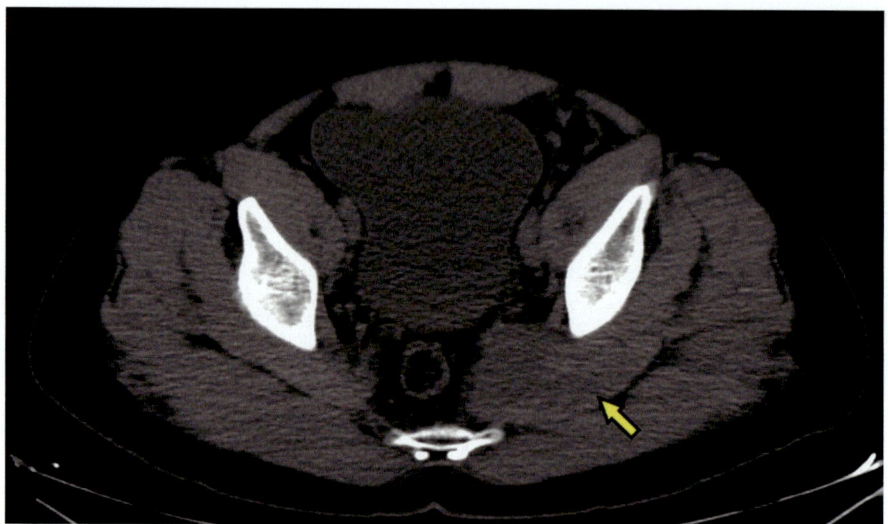

Fig. 1 Plain CT of pelvis axial section shows bulky left piriformis muscle with well-defined hypo-isodense collection

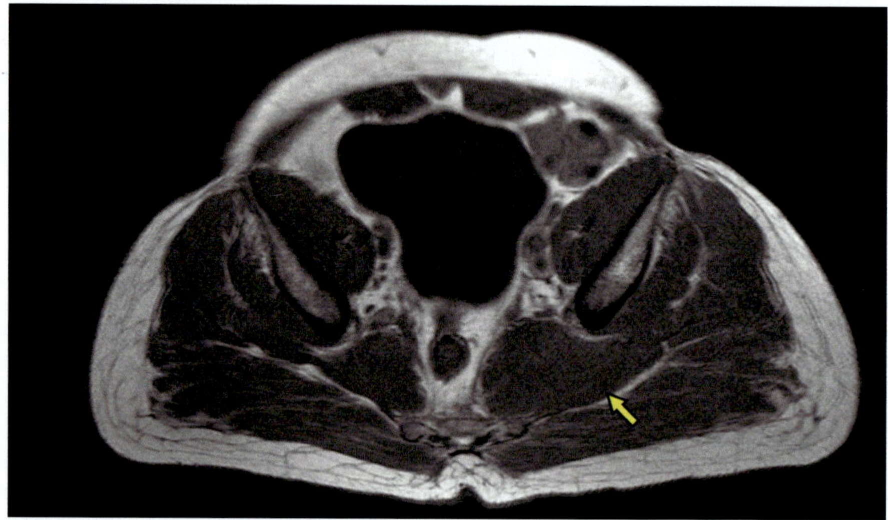

Fig. 2 MRI T1-WI of pelvis axial section shows bulky left piriformis muscle with well-defined iso-hypointense collection

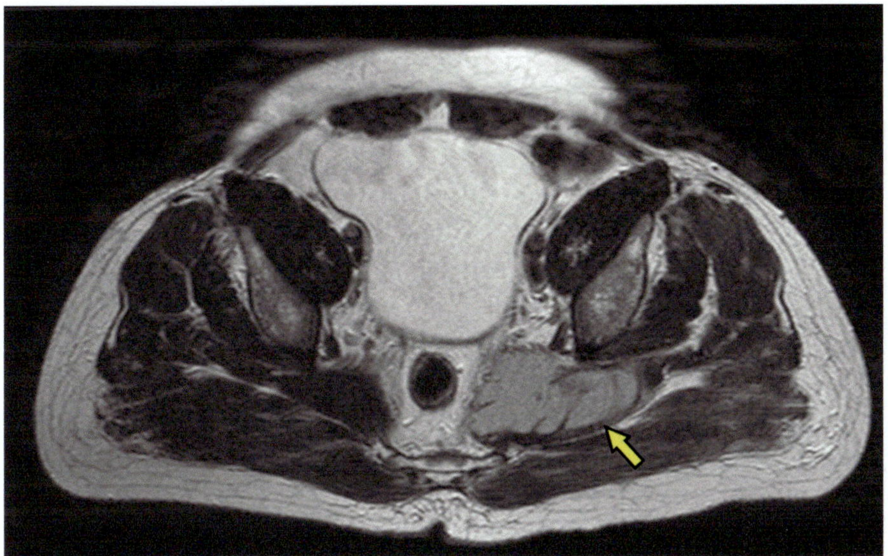

Fig. 3 MRI T2-WI of pelvis axial section shows bulky left piriformis muscle with well-defined hyperintense collection

Diffusion restriction is characteristic of abscess. STIR hyper intensity is often seen surrounding it (Fig. 4), representing edema and inflammatory changes. Post contrast T1 Fat-Sat images are useful in confirmation of abscess. The abscess shows predominantly peripheral post contrast wall enhancement with enhancing septations (Fig. 5), and hence, differentiating from malignancy- as the later show enhancing soft tissue components.

3 Discussion

The piriformis syndrome is an uncommon form of sciatic nerve neuropathy secondary to nerve entrapment (Shanmuga Jayanthan et al. 2021; Lee et al. 2004). This syndrome is characterized clinically by pain and paresthesia, in the ipsilateral gluteal region radiating into hip and posterior aspect of thigh, along the site of sciatic nerve innervation (sciatica) (Shanmuga Jayanthan et al. 2021; Lee et al. 2004). The most common cause for sciatica is lumbar disk herniation (Ergun and Lakadamyali 2010). However, there are other extra-spinal causes for it and piriformis syndrome is one of them, which accounts for only 6% of cases (Ergun and Lakadamyali 2010). Pyomyositis of piriformis muscle is a rare cause for this syndrome (Siddiq and Rasker 2019).

On clinical examination, Pace's test (pain on resisted hip external rotation and abduction) and Freiberg's sign (pain with passive internal rotation of the hip) are

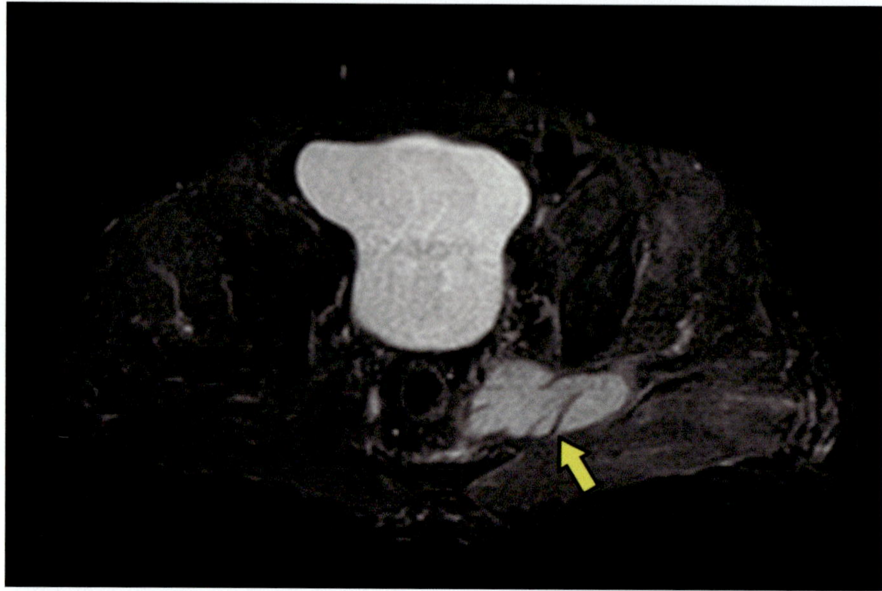

Fig. 4 MRI STIR of pelvis axial sections shows bulky left piriformis muscle with well-defined hyperintense collection. Surrounding hyperintense areas noted suggestive of edema and inflammation

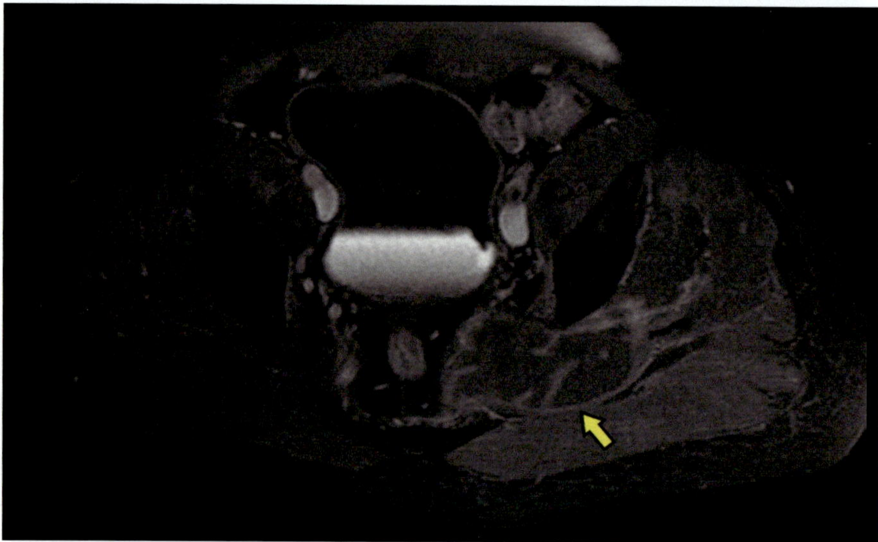

Fig. 5 MRI T1FS of contrast pelvis axial section shows predominantly peripheral post contrast wall enhancement of the collection with enhancing septations

usually positive in this piriformis syndrome. However, clinical diagnosis is difficult as the muscle is deep from palpation and symptoms are related to sciatica (Ergun and Lakadamyali 2010; Kraniotis et al. 2011).

Three different phases of inflammation are seen (Kraniotis et al. 2011). The first stage is non-purulent, where there is only mild inflammation of muscle, the second stage is characterized by pus formation (purulent stage) within muscle and third stage is identified by systemic toxicity (Kraniotis et al. 2011). The most common organism is *Staphylococcus aureus* (Kraniotis et al. 2011; Wong et al. 2008) although a single case of brucella pyomyositis is described in literature by Kraniotis et al. (2011).

The risk factors include immunocompromised status, rheumatoid arthritis, diabetes, and prior parasitic or viral infections (Kraniotis et al. 2011; Wong et al. 2008). Infections from spine and pelvis can also spread to the piriformis muscle through the endopelvic fascia (Chong and Tay 2004). Two cases of piriformis pyomyositis were reported following obstetrical interventions. It is important to diagnose this condition at early presuppurative stage, as the delay in diagnosis could result in increased morbidity and mortality.

Sciatica is a common neurological symptom, which is seen in approximately 40% of adults (Ergun and Lakadamyali 2010). It is characterized by radiating pain along the course of sciatic nerve, which is often secondary to disc degeneration that causes nerve root compression (Ergun and Lakadamyali 2010). However, there are other extra-spinal causes for sciatica, which include, trauma, infections, sacroiliitis, tumors, and so on (Ergun and Lakadamyali 2010).

Piriformis syndrome, an extra-spinal cause for sciatica, is a form of sciatic nerve entrapment neuropathy at the level of greater sciatic notch. This occurs due to piriformis muscle abnormalities like hypertrophy, inflammation, or anatomical variations (Lee et al. 2004; Ergun and Lakadamyali 2010). This syndrome accounts for only approximately 6% of all cases of sciatic neuropathy (Ergun and Lakadamyali 2010). Pyomyositis of piriformis muscle can result in piriformis syndrome, and this is a very rare cause for piriformis syndrome (Ergun and Lakadamyali 2010; Siddiq and Rasker 2019). So far, only 23 cases of piriformis pyomyositis are reported in the literature (Shanmuga Jayanthan et al. 2021; Ergun and Lakadamyali 2010).

Although contrast-enhanced CT can demonstrate intramuscular abscess with ring enhancement (Ergun and Lakadamyali 2010; Wong et al. 2008). MRI is the imaging modality of choice at early stages (presuppurative stage) due to its higher sensitivity (Shanmuga Jayanthan et al. 2021; Lee et al. 2004). Findings in MRI at early stage include enlargement of muscle with T2 and STIR hyper-intensity, without intramuscular fluid collection. Later stage, with abscess, is identified by intramuscular T1 hypointense and T2 hyper intense collection, which shows thick peripheral wall enhancement on postcontrast study (Shanmuga Jayanthan et al. 2021; Kraniotis et al. 2011). STIR hyper intensity can be seen within the muscle, suggestive of inflammatory edema.[4] Anterior displacement of the sciatic nerve with T2 signal hyper intensity may also be observed (Ergun and Lakadamyali 2010). MRI can also exclude sacroiliac joint or pelvic pathology that can result in piriformis pyomyositis (Kraniotis et al. 2011). We can also rule out disk abnormalities, which is the most common cause for sciatica (Ergun and Lakadamyali 2010; Kraniotis et al. 2011).

Treatment for myositis is intravenous antibiotics at early stages of inflammation when there is no abscess (Shanmuga Jayanthan et al. 2021; Kraniotis et al. 2011). When there is abscess formation, CT-guided or surgical drainage of abscess, along with intravenous antibiotics, is the treatment of choice (Shanmuga Jayanthan et al. 2021; Kraniotis et al. 2011). It is important to be aware of this condition as early diagnosis can significantly reduce morbidity and mortality (Kraniotis et al. 2011).

4 Conclusion

Although sciatica is commonly caused by disk pathology, it is important to get familiarized with extra-spinal causes of sciatica. Piriformis syndrome is one among the cause for extra-spinal sciatica. Piriformis pyomyositis is a rare pathology causing piriformis syndrome but has significantly high mortality, if the diagnosis is delayed. MRI has an important role to play in the early diagnosis of this condition.

References

Chong KW, Tay BK. Piriformis pyomyositis: a rare cause of sciatica. Singapore Med J. 2004;45(05):229–31.

Ergun T, Lakadamyali H. CT and MRI in the evaluation of extraspinal sciatica. Br J Radiol. 2010;83(993):791–803.

Kraniotis P, Marangos M, Lekkou A, Romanos O, Solomou E. Brucellosis presenting as piriformis myositis: a case report. J Med Case Rep. 2011;5:125.

Lee EY, Margherita AJ, Gierada DS, Narra VR. MRI of piriformis syndrome. AJR Am J Roentgenol. 2004;183(01):63–4.

Shanmuga Jayanthan S, Rajkumar SS, Kumar VS, Shalini M. Pyomyositis of the piriformis muscle—a case of piriformis syndrome. Indian J Radiol Imaging. 2021;31(4):1023–6. https://doi.org/10.1055/s-0041-1739183.PMID:35136521;PMCID:PMC8817790.

Siddiq MAB, Rasker JJ. Piriformis pyomyositis, a cause of piriformis syndrome—a systematic search and review. Clin Rheumatol. 2019;38(07):1811–21.

Wong CH, Choi SH, Wong KY. Piriformis pyomyositis: a report of three cases. J Orthop Surg (Hong Kong). 2008;16(03):389–91.

Bipartitite Piriformis Giving Rise to Sciatic Nerve Entrapment

Himanshu Agrawal, Aradhna Shukla, and Mrinal Joshi

Piriformis syndrome is a lesser-known condition that can cause pain in the buttocks, often accompanied by leg pain. It was first described in 1928 by Yeomen. The primary symptom is buttock pain, with or without leg pain, worsened by sitting or lower limb activity. Other common findings include pain in the buttocks extending from the sacrum to the greater trochanter, tenderness of the piriformis muscle during a rectal or pelvic examination, and worsening of symptoms with prolonged hip flexion, adduction, and internal rotation, in the absence of low back or hip issues. Additionally, leg length discrepancy, weak hip abductors, and pain during resisted hip abduction while sitting may also be present. Piriformis syndrome may be caused by pressure on the sciatic nerve by the piriformis muscle, and myofascial involvement of related muscles and lumbar facet syndromes may also be present.

A definitive diagnosis of piriformis syndrome is primarily based on clinical evaluation, as no conclusive diagnostic tests have been reported. In general, bone scans and electrodiagnostic studies are not helpful, although there have been a few isolated reports of their usefulness.

Bipartite piriformis syndrome is a rare variation of piriformis syndrome that can cause pain and other symptoms in the buttock and down the leg. In this condition, the piriformis muscle is divided into two parts, and the sciatic nerve passes between them, resulting in compression of the sciatic nerve and symptoms like those of classic

H. Agrawal (✉)
Department of Physical Medicine and Rehabilitation, All India Institute of Medical Sciences, Jodhpur, Rajasthan, India
e-mail: drhimanshuagrawal86@gmail.com

A. Shukla
Pain and Palliative Fellow, Department of Physical Medicine and Rehabilitation, AIIMS, Jodhpur, All India Institute of Medical Sciences, Jodhpur, Rajasthan, India

M. Joshi
Department of Physical Medicine and Rehabilitation, SMS Medical College and Associated Hospitals, Jaipur, Rajasthan, India

© The Author(s), under exclusive license to Springer Nature Switzerland AG 2023 47
K. M. Iyer (ed.), *Piriformis Syndrome*,
https://doi.org/10.1007/978-3-031-40736-9_12

piriformis syndrome. Diagnosing bipartite piriformis syndrome can be challenging and requires careful evaluation of imaging studies such as MRI or CT scans. Treatment options include conservative measures such as stretching, physical therapy, and anti-inflammatory medications, and in severe cases, injection therapy or surgical intervention may be necessary.

It is essential to note that bipartite piriformis syndrome is rare, and most cases are not associated with this anatomical variation. If you are experiencing buttock or leg pain symptoms or suspect that you have piriformis syndrome (Hopayian and Danielyan 2010; Pecina and Bojanic 2008; Lutz and Burkhard 2021).

1 Epidemiology

Entrapment of the sciatic nerve by the piriformis nowadays has become a common diagnosis due to the emergence of high- quality case studies and evidence showing a prevalence of anatomic variation between the piriformis and sciatic nerve (Figs. 1, 2, and 3).

The anatomical variations of the piriformis and sciatic nerve found were described following Beaton and Anton's classification. As we understand this classification, true bipartite piriformis falls in types B (Fig. 2), D & E of the above classification.

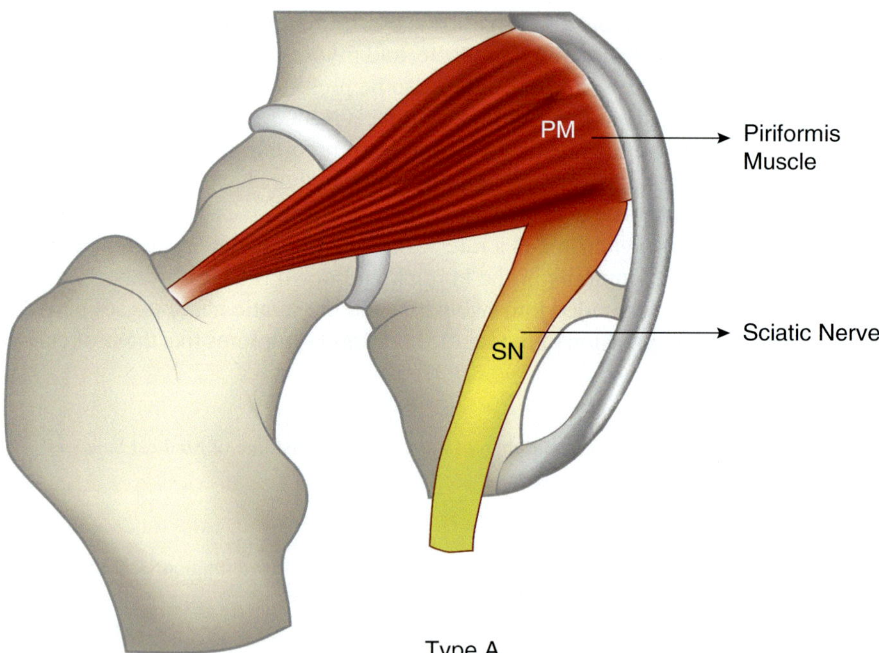

Fig. 1 Beaton and Anton's classification type A

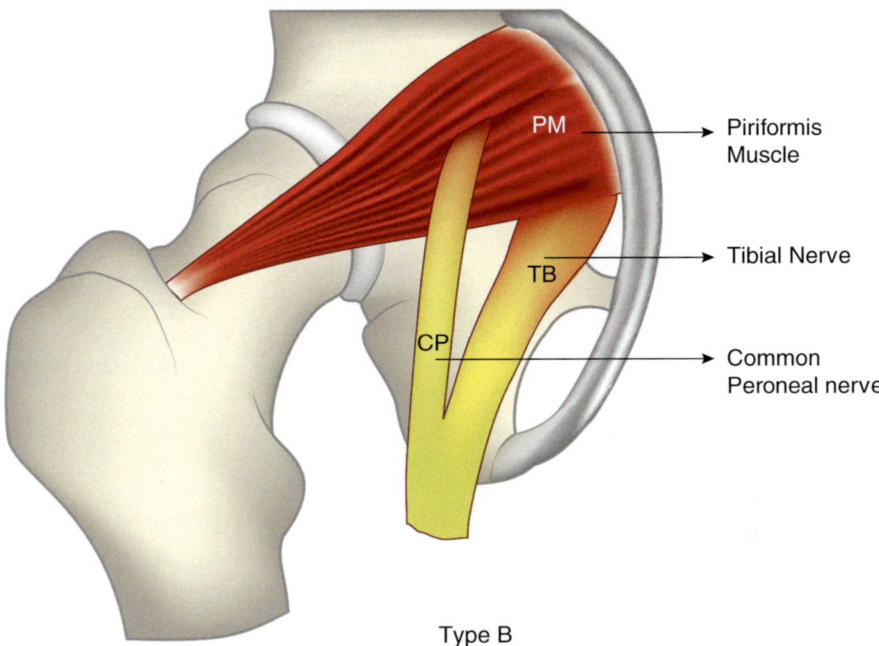

Fig. 2 Beaton and Anton's classification type B

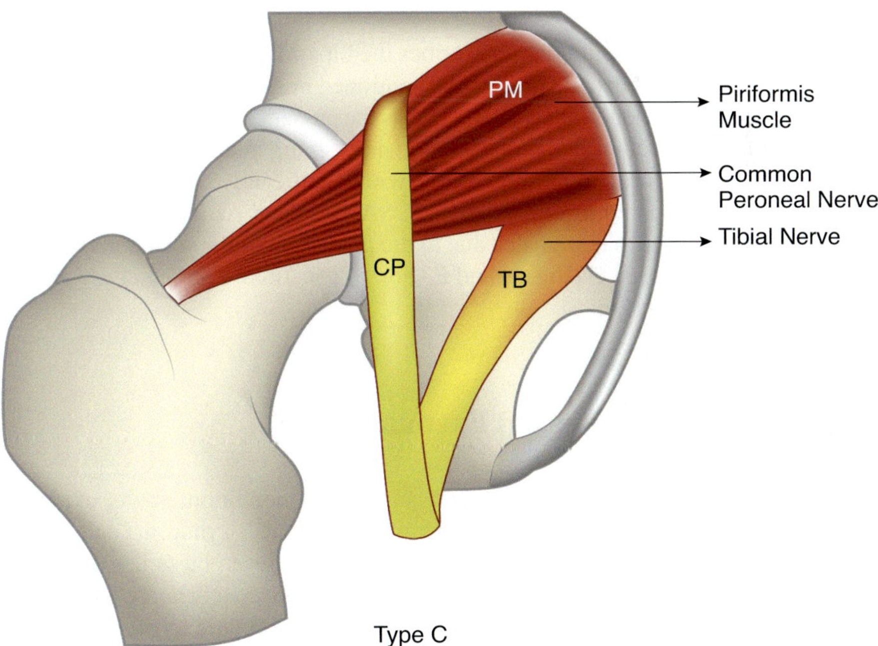

Fig. 3 Beaton and Anton's classification type C

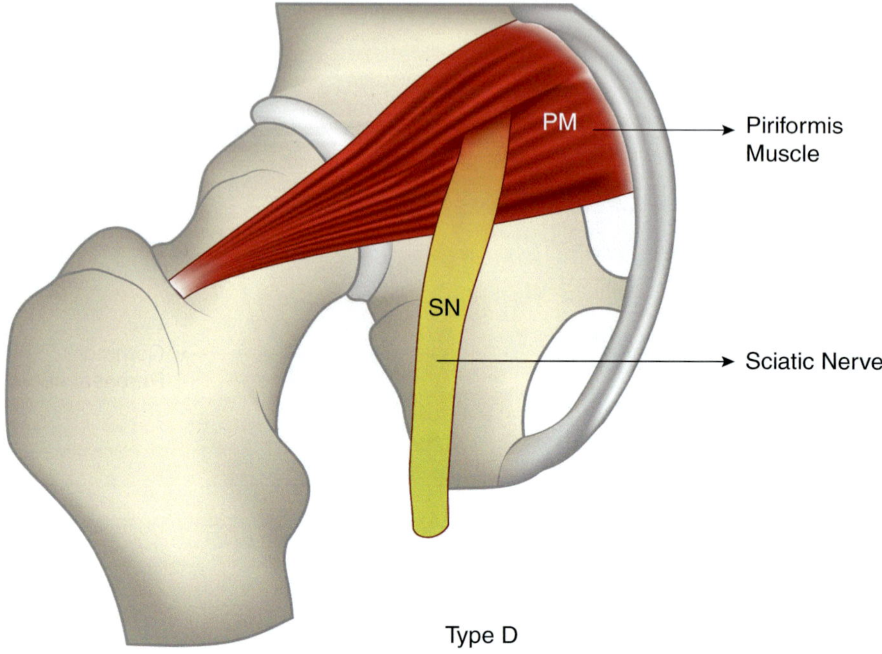

Fig. 4 Beaton and Anton's classification type D

No other classification singularly describes the bipartite piriformis alone, considering the prevalence of bipartite piriformis mentioned in studies using the classification mentioned above, states that type B which is the passage of one division of sciatic nerve through and the other division of sciatic nerve lying anteriorly to the bipartite piriformis muscle has around 8% prevalence with significantly higher prevalence in east Asia (24%) compared to Europe (9%), USA (4%) and Africa (3%). Type B is more prevalent in females than males due to the proximity of the sciatic nerve to the reproductive organs. Type D (Fig. 4) and E (Fig. 5) constitute ever lesser prevalence in the population (1%) (Fig. 6).

2 Clinical Presentation and Examination

The bipartite piriformis is an uncommon anatomical condition, so its existence does not cause any novel symptoms. Symptoms of piriformis syndrome and lumbar vertebra diseases are very similar, and differentiation between these is often tricky (Kosukegawa et al. 1976). All the findings corroborate the sciatic nerve entrapment picture like pain spreading from the buttocks through the sciatic territory radiating

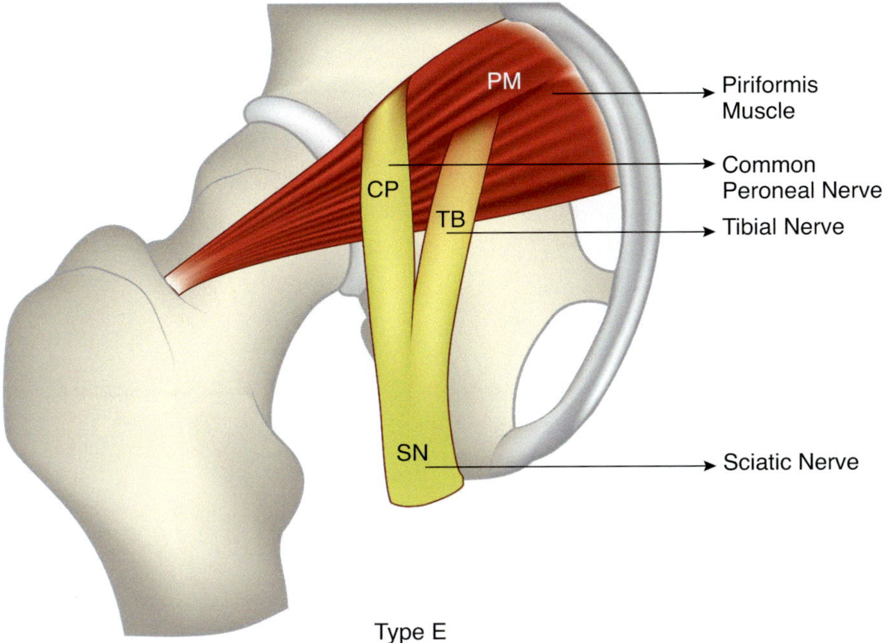

Fig. 5 Beaton and Anton's classification type E

down the limb. The intensity might vary along with some specific aggravating conditions that might or not be present. Aggravating conditions might be sitting on a hard surface or sitting cross- legged.

Localisation of the condition can be confirmed by elicitation of exact symptoms, i.e., radiating pain to the lower leg by pressure over the piriformis muscle and passive internal rotation of the hip inducing radiating pain to the lower leg Freiberg's sign (Freiberg and Vinke 1934) also Pace's test (Frost 1881) i.e., pain and weakness with resisted hip external rotation and abduction. The different manoeuvers aim to reproduce the pain experienced by the patient: buttock pain and sciatic tingling or numbness in the limb affected and accompanied in some cases by distal paresthesia (Kosukegawa et al. 1976). Other special tests that can be applied are Beatty's maneuver (Beatty 1994) and Fishman's FAIR test (Flexion—Adduction—Internal Rotation test) (Fishman et al. 2002). But a high degree of clinical suspicion is needed to diagnose the condition solely on special tests as none of these particular tests has been validated for specificity and sensitivity (Steiner et al. 1987). Pace's test and Freiberg's sign were reported to be present in only 65% of patients (Michel et al. 2013). A definitive diagnosis is often impossible because of the lack of an established imaging method for image diagnosis.

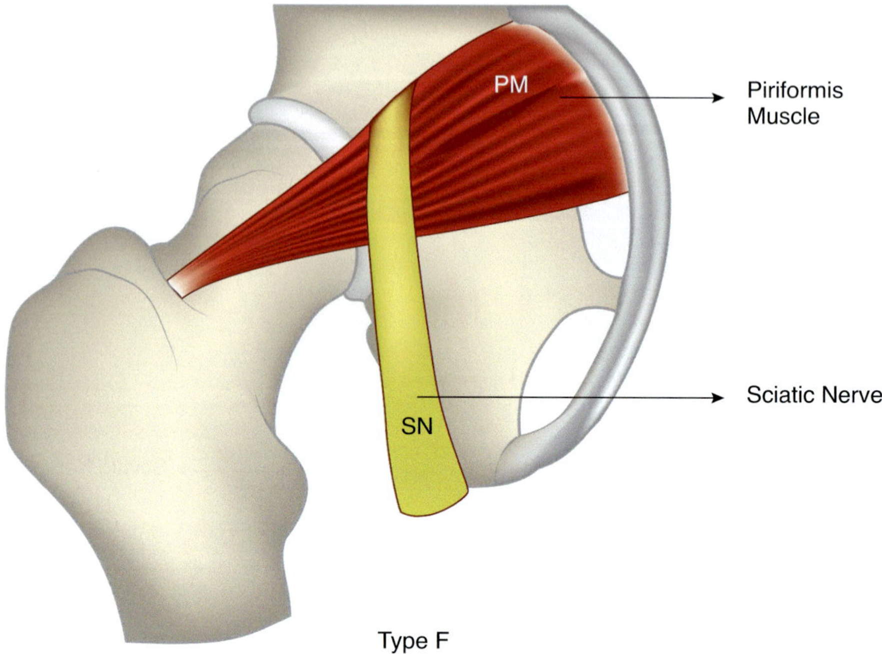

Fig. 6 Beaton and Anton's classification type F

3 Diagnosis

Sciatic nerve entrapment is an elusive clinical entity itself. Bipartite Piriformis is eventually an anatomical extraspinal cause of sciatic nerve entrapment. Its mere presence does not indicate sciatic nerve entrapment. As described in the earlier section, a high index of clinical suspicion is needed to determine the concerned condition, which means ruling out all the other causes that can mimic sciatic nerve entrapment. Systematic clinical assessment will generally lead to the correct diagnosis. Apart from that, when a differential of extraspinal sciatica is in play, imaging comes in handy. Dynamic scans can be beneficial in the clinical scenario. With the emergence of musculoskeletal USG usage in pain clinics or rehabilitation facilities, piriformis muscle anomalies can be easily demonstrated.

A definitive diagnosis is often impossible because of the need for an established imaging method for image diagnosis. Apart from musculoskeletal USG, Pelvic MRI (Fig. 7) and peri neurography of the sciatic nerve followed by CT is very useful for determining the anatomic association between the piriformis muscle and the sciatic nerve (Kosukegawa et al. 2006). There have been a few reports on the prediction of anatomic variation based on findings of hypertrophy of the piriformis muscle obtained by using pelvic CT and MRI (Pamela 1991; Ozaki et al. 1999; Paolo et al. 2001).

One can use the proposed algorithm by the authors to establish the condition.

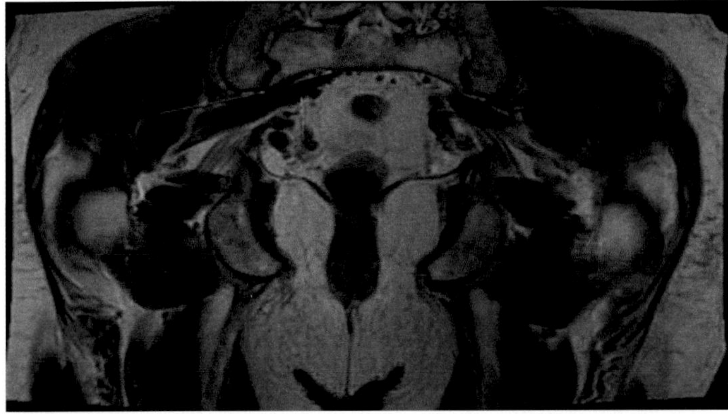

Fig. 7 Showing coronal section of Male pelvis bi partite piriformis muscle. The piriformis is identified with a green arrow. (Joshi M, Agrawal H, Sukhani P. Bipartite piriformis: a rare case of sciatic nerve entrapment. Int. J. Heal. Clin. Res. [Internet]. 2020 Nov.10];3(9):45–8.)

4 Differential Diagnosis

The symptoms of piriformis syndrome can be like those of other conditions, and a proper differential diagnosis is essential to ensure the appropriate treatment is administered. Here are some situations that may be considered in the differential diagnosis of piriformis syndrome, along with references for further information:

A. Deep gluteal syndrome: Obturator internus and Gemelli complex might also be potential causes of neural compression. Pain arising in the buttock and hamstring region can also indicate entrapment of the posterior cutaneous nerve of the thigh rather than the sciatic nerve alone (Filler et al. 2005).
B. Sciatic Notch Syndrome: Sciatic nerve entrapment in the ischial tunnel adjoining hamstring muscle attachment mimics the symptom of piriformis syndrome.
C. Wallet neuritis/Fat wallet Syndrome: Placement of the patient's wallet in the back pocket of their attire, precisely behind the piriformis muscle, has the potential to constrict the sciatic nerve on the same side (Siddiq et al. 2018).
D. Lumbar radiculopathy: This condition involves compression of the spinal nerves in the lower back, which can cause pain, numbness, and weakness in the buttock and legs. It can sometimes be difficult to distinguish from piriformis syndrome, but a thorough physical exam and diagnostic imaging can help differentiate between the two conditions (Maugars et al. 1996).
E. Sacroiliac joint dysfunction: Dysfunction of the sacroiliac joint, which connects the sacrum to the pelvis, can cause pain in the lower back, buttock, and leg. This condition may be considered in the differential diagnosis of piriformis syndrome (Bernard and Kirkaldy-Willis 1987).
F. Ischial bursitis: Inflammation of the ischial bursa, a fluid-filled sac near the sit bones in the buttock, can cause pain radiating down the leg and is sometimes mistaken for piriformis syndrome (Regan and Cohen 2010).

G. Spinal tumors: Although rare, tumors in the spine or surrounding tissues can compress the sciatic nerve, leading to symptoms resembling piriformis syndrome.

H. Hamstring muscle tear: A tear in one of the hamstring muscles can cause pain in the buttock region, similar to the pain experienced in piriformis syndrome.

I. Hamstring tendonitis: Hamstring tendonitis involves inflammation of the tendons at the back of the thigh, near the buttock region. It can cause pain and tenderness in the area, which may resemble the symptoms of piriformis syndrome.

5 Treatment Algorithm

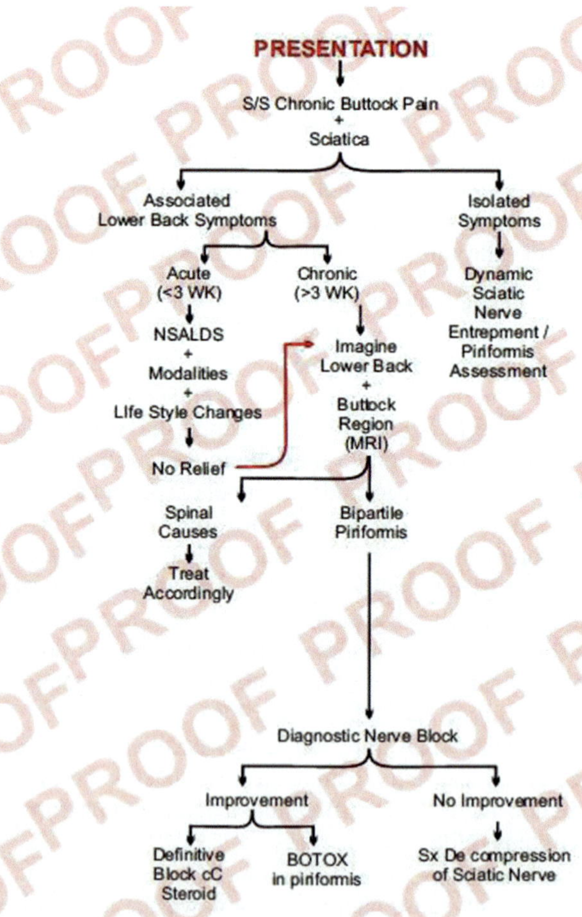

6 Treatment

The disease must be approached conservatively in the early stages of the symptomatic bipartite piriformis, i.e., clinically sciatic nerve entrapment. The prescription of NSAIDs, dynamic stretching of the piriformis muscle, and modalities such as iontophoresis should be started. If unresponsive to conservative management, targeted intervention like USG-guided steroid injection or Botox can be taken up (Cass 2015).

For recalcitrant cases piriformis tenotomy and decompression of the sciatic nerve can be done (Cass 2015; Dezawa et al. 2003). Case reports have been published where arthroscopically release of piriformis muscle was done for definitive treatment (Pierce et al. 2017) as well case reports were published for resection of the anterior and posterior lobe of piriformis muscle for type D Beaton's variant (Kosukegawa et al. 1976).

References

Beatty RA. The piriformis muscle syndrome: a simple diagnostic maneuver. Neurosurgery 1994;34:512–4 View in References Cross Reference.

Bernard TN Jr, Kirkaldy-Willis WH. Recognising specific characteristics of nonspecific low back pain. Clin Orthop Relat Res. 1987;217:266–80.

Cass SP. Piriformis syndrome: a cause of non-discogenic sciatica. Curr Sports Med Rep. 2015;14(1):41–4. https://doi.org/10.1249/JSR.0000000000000110. PMID: 25574881.

Dezawa A, Kusano S, Miki H. Arthroscopic release of the piriformis muscle under local anesthesia for piriformis syndrome. Arthroscopy. 2003;19(5):554–7. https://doi.org/10.1053/jars.2003.50158. PMID: 12724687.

Filler AG, Haynes J, Jordan SE, Prager J, Villablanca JP, Farahani K, Mcbride DQ, Tsuruda JS, Morisoli B, Batzdorf U, Johnson JP. Sciatica of non-disc origin and piriformis syndrome: diagnosis by magnetic resonance neurography and interventional magnetic resonance imaging with outcome study of resulting treatment. J Neurosurg Spine. 2005;2(2):99–115.

Fishman LM, Dombi GW, Michaelsen C, Ringel SV, Rosbruch J, Rosner B, et al. Piriformis syndrome: diagnosis, treatment, and outcome—a 10-year study. Arch Phys Med Rehabil. 2002;83:295–301.

Freiberg AH, Vinke TA. Sciatica and the sacro-iliac joint. J Bone Joint Surg Am. 1934;16:126–36.

Frost JJ. Contribution à l'étude clinique de la sciatique. Paris: University of Paris; 1881.

Hopayian K, Danielyan A. Four symptoms define the piriformis syndrome: an updated systematic review of its clinical features. Eur J Orthop Surg Traumatol. 2010;20(8):565–71.

Joshi M, Agrawal H, Sukhani P. Bipartite piriformis: a rare case of sciatic nerve entrapment. Int J Heal Clin Res. [Internet]. 2020;3(9):45–8.

Kosukegawa I, Yoshimoto M, Isogai S, Nonaka S, Yamashita T. Piriformis syndrome resulting from a rare anatomic variation. Spine (Phila Pa 1976). 2006;31(18):E664–6. https://doi.org/10.1097/01.brs.0000231877.34800.71. PMID: 16915082.

Kosukegawa I, Yoshimoto M, Isogai S, Nonaka S, Yamashita T. Piriformis syndrome resulting from a rare anatomic variation. Spine 2006;31(18):E664–6. https://doi.org/10.1097/01.brs.0000231877.34800.71

Lutz AM, Burkhard A. Bipartite piriformis muscle syndrome: a review of the literature. Cureus. 2021;13(8): e18089.

Maugars Y, Mathis C, Berthelot JM, Charlier C, Prost A. Assessment of the diagnostic value of the medical history and physical examination for common lumbar spine complaints. Arthritis Rheum. 1996;39(4):663–70.

Michel F, Decavel P, Toussirot E, Tatu L, Aleton E, Monnier G, Garbuio P, Parratte B. The piriformis muscle syndrome: an exploration of anatomical context, pathophysiological hypotheses and diagnostic criteria. Ann Phys Rehabil Med. 2013;56(4):300–11. https://doi.org/10.1016/j.rehab.2013.03.006. Epub 2013 Apr 30. PMID: 23684469.

Ozaki S, Hamabe T, Muro T. Piriformis syndrome resulting from an anomalous relationship between the sciatic nerve and piriformis muscle. Orthopedics 1999;22:771–2.

Pamela MB. Piriformis syndrome: a rational approach to management. Pain 1991;47:345–52.

Paolo R, Patrizio C, Marano S. Magnetic resonance imaging findings in piriformis syndrome: a case report. Arch Phys Med Rehabil. 2001;82:519–21.

Pecina M, Bojanic I. The piriformis syndrome–myth or reality? Coll Antropol. 2008;32(1):293–7.

Pierce TP, Pierce CM, Issa K, McInerney VK, Festa A, Scillia AJ. Arthroscopic piriformis release–a technique for sciatic nerve decompression 2017. https://doi.org/10.1016/j.eats.2016.09.012. PMID: 28409095; PMCID: PMC5382232.

Regan WD, Cohen MJ. Ischiogluteal bursitis: a report of two cases and a literature review. Clin Orthop Relat Res. 2010;468(10):2695–8.

Siddiq MA, Jahan I, Masih Uzzaman SA. Wallet neuritis–an example of peripheral sensitization. Curr Rheumatol Rev. 2018;14(3):279–83.

Steiner C, Staubs C, Ganon M, et al. Piriformis syndrome: pathogenesis, diagnosis and treatment. J Am Osteopath Assoc. 1987;87:318–23.

Hydrodissection of Piriformis Syndrome

Mihiro Kaga

1 Introduction

Hydrodissection is a kind of injection therapy that aims to mechanically separate the target structure from the surrounding structures and decompress it (Buntragulpoontawee et al. 2021). Piriformis syndrome is caused by compression of the sciatic nerve; pathologies that contribute to its development include anatomic abnormalities of the sciatic nerve and piriformis muscle (Natsis et al. 2014), piriformis muscle injury due to trauma (Robinson 1947), piriformis muscle hypertrophy (Russell et al. 2008), and piriformis muscle spasm (Fishman et al. 2002). Furthermore, adhesions between the piriformis muscle and tissues surrounding the sciatic nerve, which runs proximal to the pisiform muscle, have been reported to have a significant impact on piriformis syndrome (Shah et al. 2019; Benson and Schutzer 1999; Haghnegahdar et al. 2015). Thus, there are various pathological conditions that contribute to the development of piriformis syndrome. I argue that the pathological condition of adhesions, especially those caused by surrounding tissues, could be treated by hydrodissection; this is the first study to reports the first case of piriformis syndrome treated by ultrasound-guided hydrodissection in this series of cases (Kaga and Ueda 2022a, b). I, the author, am a Japanese general practitioner who treats patients from all departments and practices in a variety of fields, from remote island clinics to emergency centers. This section outlines the actual treatment of hydrodissection as practiced in my clinical practice.

M. Kaga (✉)
Department of Clinical Biostatistics, Graduate School of Medical and Dental Sciences,
Tokyo Medical and Dental University, Tokyo, Japan
e-mail: mihirokaga@gmail.com

2 Indication

As mentioned previously, hydrodissection is considered when the pathogenesis of pisiform muscle syndrome is thought to be related to the pathology of adhesions from surrounding tissues. I emphasize the relevance of Myofascial Pain Syndrome (MPS) as a background for the pathology of adhesions from surrounding tissues and other pathologies that contribute to the development of the syndrome (Kaga and Ueda 2022a). Thus, hydrodissection is a good indication for piriformis syndrome when it is presumed to be caused by a pathology related to MPS. The musculoskeletal condition known as MPS is believed to originate from localized, taut regions consisting of skeletal muscle and fascia, which are referred to as trigger points (Wheeler 2004). The causes of MPS are varied, including muscle damage, overuse, and spasm, and may involve complex pathologies other than the adhesion pathology reported in our case series (Money 2017; Galasso et al. 2020). The identification of a myofascial trigger point and its correlation with the patient's pain complaint is crucial for diagnosing MPS. To identify a myofascial trigger point, palpation is performed (Gerwin 2014). The myofascial trigger point has three essential features for diagnosis, including a taut band within the muscle, exquisite tenderness at a point on the taut band, and reproduction of the patient's pain, while the last five features such as local twitch response, referred pain, weakness, restricted range of motion, and autonomic signs are not necessary for diagnosis (Gerwin 2014). Range of motion can also be evaluated with ultrasound. Ultrasonography of the bilateral piriformis muscles with internal or external rotation of the hip joint can assess the sliding of the piriformis muscle, range of motion, and the existence of adhesions, as this muscle plays a crucial role in the external rotation of the hip joint (Battaglia et al. 2016). It is easier to determine the indication for hydrodissection if the patient is examined with the MPS diagnostic method in mind when taking a history and conducting a physical examination.

3 Procedure

Hydrodissection is performed under ultrasound guidance to ensure that the injection is administered at the targeted site. The patient is placed in the supine position and the piriformis muscle is visualized using a convex probe (Fig. 1).

In lean patients, a linear probe can also be used to delineate the piriformis muscle, and the resolution of the image is better than that of a convex probe. Since the piriformis muscle arises from the anterior surface of the sacrum and is inserted into the greater trochanter (Probst et al. 2019), it is easier to identify the piriformis muscle by recognizing these landmarks on the body surface and then applying the probe. Once the piriformis muscle is identified, the sciatic nerve running through the infrapiriform foramen is also identified to prevent complications from accidental puncture; the inferior gluteal artery and vein are also identified by applying color doppler (Fig. 2).

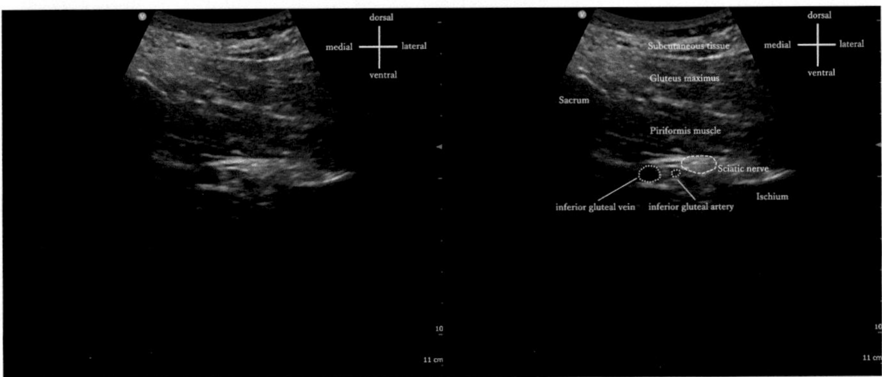

Fig. 1 Drawing of the piriformis muscle (the modality used was Vscan Air, GE Healthcare Japan Corporation, Tokyo, Japan)

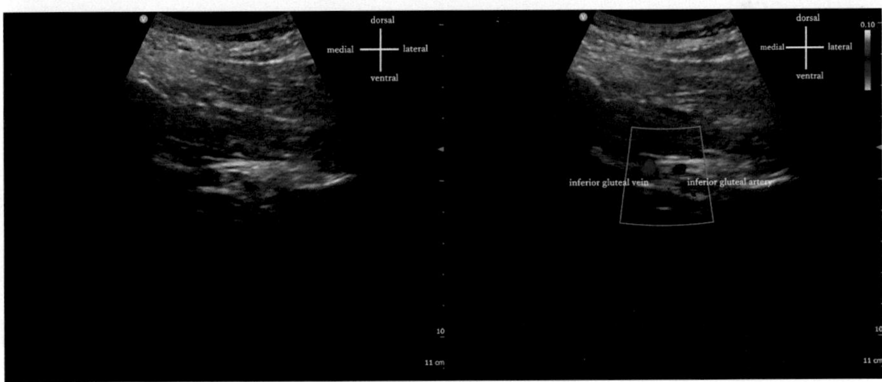

Fig. 2 Drawing of the inferior gluteal artery and vein by color doppler imaging

Then, using a Cathelin needle (e.g., 23G60 mm), the in- or out-of-plane technique is used to inject the drug into the deep layer of the piriformis muscle (Fig. 3).

I often inject a total of 10–20 mL of a solution consisting of 1 mL of 1% lidocaine and 9 mL of saline, but the effect is also observed with the saline/lactate Ringer's solution alone without using a local anesthetic. In Japan, I mix a very small amount of local anesthetic with the saline/lactate Ringer's solution for injection because the insurance does not allow the injection of saline/lactate Ringer's solution alone.

Additionally, I have recently been using mobile handheld ultrasound to perform injection therapy. GE HealthCare's Vscan Air (Fig. 4) can be linked to a hand-held iPhone or iPad to view high-quality ultrasound images. The Vscan Air is small and lightweight (131 mm high, 64 mm wide, and 205 g in weight) and can be activated quickly, making it highly mobile and recommended for use in busy outpatient clinics.

The disadvantage of the Vscan Air is that it has a short continuous use time of approximately 50 min and needs to be recharged quickly. The price is approximately 1 million Japanese yen. Of course I declare no conflicts of interest associated with this manuscript.

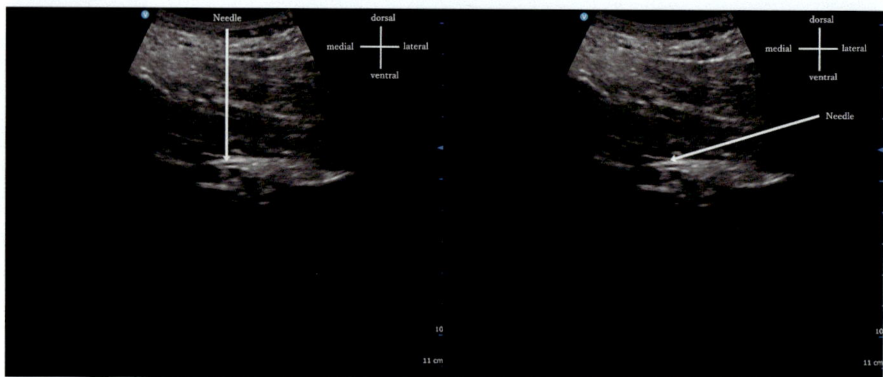

Fig. 3 Ultrasound image at the time of puncture (in- or out-of-plane technique)

Fig. 4 Vscan Air, the author's favorite mobile handheld ultrasound

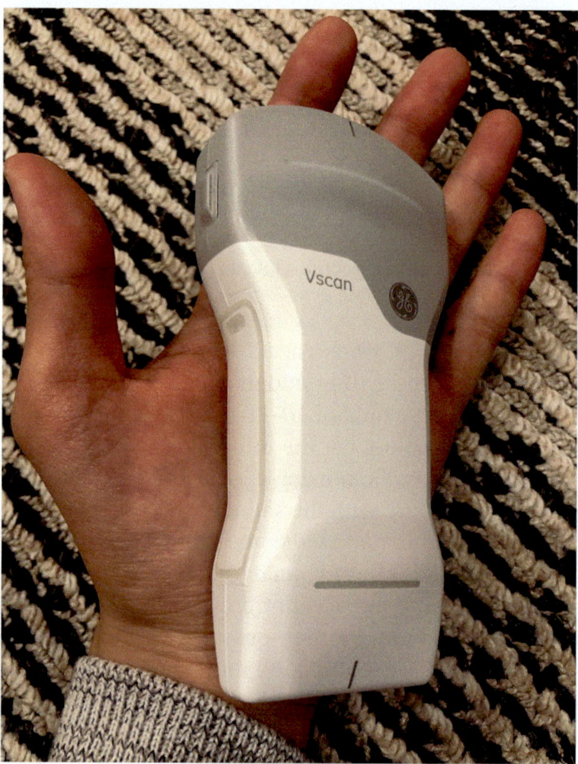

4 Therapy Evaluation

If piriformis syndrome is the background of the MPS-related pathology, the effect is often seen immediately after the injection. In my experience, many patients have reported the disappearance of pain or have been able to walk without pain immediately after the injection. If there is no change in symptoms 15 min after injection, I consider that the injection was ineffective and reevaluate the diagnosis. Thus, hydrodissection has a diagnostic treatment aspect because the effect of the treatment is immediately apparent. If injections are administered only with saline/lactate Ringer's solution, the adverse events of local anesthetic poisoning (Gitman et al. 2019) associated with local anesthetic administration do not occur in the first place. The risk of accidental puncture (Greensmith and Murray 2006) is low because the puncture is made under ultrasound guidance, making it a less invasive treatment. For these reasons, hydrodissection can be aggressively performed in patients with piriformis syndrome in whom the pathophysiology of pain is unknown.

5 Follow up

Even when injections are effective, symptoms may recur during the acute phase; thus, follow-up should be conducted every week, and in some cases, injections are administered again. NSAIDs and acetaminophen are often prescribed to deal with recurrent pain at home. Furthermore, piriformis syndrome is often caused by repetitive movements in the patient's daily life that place repetitive stress on the piriformis muscle. Identification of the causative movements, followed by lifestyle guidance and physical therapy (Gulledge et al. 2014), is the most important part of treatment, and should be done concurrently with injection therapy. With a combination of these treatments, piriformis syndrome will heal and injections will gradually become unnecessary.

6 Future Development

Hydrodissection for MPS-related pathology is not only effective for piriformis syndrome, but can also be applied to other diseases, since MPS can occur anywhere in the body. The author was the first to report cases of hydrodissection being effective for headache (occipital neuralgia) and abdominal pain (ventral ramus of spinal nerve entrapment syndrome (VERNES)) (Kaga 2022a, b). Hydrodissection is thus a versatile and highly effective therapeutic technique that improves symptoms immediately after injection and is highly satisfactory for patients. I would be more than happy if more readers develop an interest in hydrodissection after reading this section.

References

Battaglia PJ, Mattox R, Haun DW, Welk AB, Kettner NW. Dynamic ultrasonography of the deep external rotator musculature of the hip: a descriptive study. PM R. 2016;8(7):640–50. https://doi.org/10.1016/j.pmrj.2015.11.001. Epub 2015 Nov 10. PMID: 26548967.

Benson ER, Schutzer SF. Posttraumatic piriformis syndrome: diagnosis and results of operative treatment. J Bone Joint Surg Am. 1999;81(7):941–9. PMID: 10428125.

Buntragulpoontawee M, Chang KV, Vitoonpong T, Pornjaksawan S, Kitisak K, Saokaew S, et al. The effectiveness and safety of commonly used injectates for ultrasound-guided hydrodissection treatment of peripheral nerve entrapment syndromes: a systematic review. Front Pharmacol. 2021;11: 621150. https://doi.org/10.3389/fphar.2020.621150.PMID:33746745;PMCID: PMC7973278.

Fishman LM, Anderson C, Rosner B. BOTOX and physical therapy in the treatment of piriformis syndrome. Am J Phys Med Rehabil. 2002;81(12):936–42. https://doi.org/10.1097/00002060-200212000-00009. PMID: 12447093.

Galasso A, Urits I, An D, Nguyen D, Borchart M, Yazdi C, et al. A comprehensive review of the treatment and management of myofascial pain syndrome. Curr Pain Headache Rep. 2020;24(8):43. https://doi.org/10.1007/s11916-020-00877-5. PMID: 32594264.

Gerwin RD. Diagnosis of myofascial pain syndrome. Phys Med Rehabil Clin N Am. 2014;25(2):341–55. https://doi.org/10.1016/j.pmr.2014.01.011. Epub 2014 Mar 18. PMID: 24787337.

Gitman M, Fettiplace MR, Weinberg GL, Neal JM, Barrington MJ. Local anesthetic systemic toxicity: a narrative literature review and clinical update on prevention, diagnosis, and management. Plast Reconstr Surg. 2019;144(3):783–95. https://doi.org/10.1097/PRS.000000000000 5989. PMID: 31461049.

Greensmith JE, Murray WB. Complications of regional anesthesia. Curr Opin Anaesthesiol. 2006;19(5):531–7. https://doi.org/10.1097/01.aco.0000245280.99786.a3. PMID: 16960487.

Gulledge BM, Marcellin-Little DJ, Levine D, Tillman L, Harrysson OL, Osborne JA, et al. Comparison of two stretching methods and optimization of stretching protocol for the piriformis muscle. Med Eng Phys. 2014;36(2):212–8. https://doi.org/10.1016/j.medengphy.2013.10.016. Epub 2013 Nov 19. PMID: 24262799.

Haghnegahdar A, Sedighi M, Motalebi H. Piriformis muscle syndrome: a recurrent case after surgical release. J Surg Case Rep. 2015;2015(8):rjv105. https://doi.org/10.1093/jscr/rjv105. PMID: 26286539; PMCID: PMC4539510.

Kaga M. First case of occipital neuralgia treated by fascial hydrodissection. Am J Case Rep. 2022a;23:e936475. https://doi.org/10.12659/AJCR.936475. PMID: 35578561; PMCID: PMC9125529.

Kaga M. A case report on abdominal pain treated with a new technique of ultrasound-guided transversus abdominis plane hydrodissection using a low concentration of local anesthetics. Cureus. 2022b;14(11):e31966. https://doi.org/10.7759/cureus.31966. PMID: 36582553; PMCID: PMC9795083.

Kaga M, Ueda T. Effectiveness of hydro-dissection of the piriformis muscle plus low-dose local anesthetic injection for piriformis syndrome: a report of 2 cases. Am J Case Rep. 2022a;23: e935346. https://doi.org/10.12659/AJCR.935346.PMID:35124689;PMCID:PMC8829885.

Kaga M, Ueda T. Errate: effectiveness of hydro-dissection of the piriformis muscle plus low-dose local anesthetic injection for piriformis syndrome: a report of 2 cases. Am J Case Rep. 2022b;23: e938966. https://doi.org/10.12659/AJCR.938966.Erratumfor:AmJCaseRep.23: e935346.PMID:36408596;PMCID:PMC9703950.

Money S. Pathophysiology of trigger points in myofascial pain syndrome. J Pain Palliat Care Pharmacother. 2017;31(2):158–9. https://doi.org/10.1080/15360288.2017.1298688. Epub 2017 Apr 5. PMID: 28379050.

Natsis K, Totlis T, Konstantinidis GA, Paraskevas G, Piagkou M, Koebke J. Anatomical variations between the sciatic nerve and the piriformis muscle: a contribution to surgical anatomy in piriformis syndrome. Surg Radiol Anat. 2014;36(3):273–80. https://doi.org/10.1007/s00276-013-1180-7. Epub 2013 Jul 31. PMID: 23900507.

Probst D, Stout A, Hunt D. Piriformis syndrome: a narrative review of the anatomy, diagnosis, and treatment. PM R. 2019;11 Suppl 1:S54–63. https://doi.org/10.1002/pmrj.12189. Epub 2019 Jul 22. PMID: 31102324.

Robinson DR. Pyriformis syndrome in relation to sciatic pain. Am J Surg. 1947;73(3):355–8. https://doi.org/10.1016/0002-9610(47)90345-0. PMID: 20289074.

Russell JM, Kransdorf MJ, Bancroft LW, Peterson JJ, Berquist TH, Bridges MD. Magnetic resonance imaging of the sacral plexus and piriformis muscles. Skeletal Radiol. 2008;37(8):709–13. https://doi.org/10.1007/s00256-008-0486-8. Epub 2008 Jun 3. PMID: 18521595.

Shah SS, Consuegra JM, Subhawong TK, Urakov TM, Manzano GR. Epidemiology and etiology of secondary piriformis syndrome: a single-institution retrospective study. J Clin Neurosci. 2019;59:209–12. https://doi.org/10.1016/j.jocn.2018.10.069. Epub 2018 Oct 24. PMID: 30528358.

Wheeler AH. Myofascial pain disorders: theory to therapy. Drugs 2004;64(1):45–62. https://doi.org/10.2165/00003495-200464010-00004. PMID: 14723558.

Composite Anatomical Variations Between the Sciatic Nerve and the Piriformis Muscle

Ameet Kumar Jha, Samal Nauhria, Dheeraj Bansal, Praghosh Chhetri, and Prakash Baral

1 Introduction

Piriformis syndrome (PS) is a debilitating condition characterized by pain, numbness, and tingling sensations in the buttocks and lower extremities resulting from compression or irritation of the sciatic nerve by the piriformis muscle, a small muscle located deep within the gluteal region. The piriformis muscle functions as an external rotator of the hip and is adjacently related to the sciatic nerve. While the anatomy of the piriformis muscle and its relationship with the sciatic nerve is well-known, there are significant variations in their structure and position among individuals. These anatomical variations can contribute to the development and clinical presentation of PS (Hicks et al. 2023). This chapter aims to comprehend the variations of the piriformis muscle and sciatic nerve and their implications in the pathogenesis and management of PS.

Sciatic nerve entrapment along its course results in conditions like sciatica and PS. PS is a painful condition responsible for 6% of low back pain cases (Mitra et al. 2014; Yeoman 1928). It is one of the non-discogenic causes of sciatica resulting due to trauma, inflammation, and degenerative changes to the piriformis muscle. However, rare structural variations can be one of the main causes of this syndrome (Ro and Edmonds 2018; Natsis et al. 2014). Therefore, awareness of the anatomical variation of the sciatic nerve and piriformis muscle is essential for clinical procedures such as hip arthroplasty, sciatic nerve block, and gluteal surgery. Understanding these variations can also minimize the iatrogenic injuries resulting from these procedures (Tomaszewski et al. 2016). The structural variation of the sciatic nerve, piriformis muscle, and their relations was first classified by Beaton and Anson into six categories in 1937 (Table 1).

A. K. Jha (✉) · S. Nauhria · D. Bansal · P. Chhetri · P. Baral
Anatomical Sciences, Saint Matthews University School of Medicine, George Town, Cayman Islands
e-mail: akjha@stmatthews.edu

Table 1 Beaton and Anson classification (Beaton and Anson 1937)

Type a	Undivided nerve below the undivided muscle
Type b	Divisions of the nerve between and below the undivided muscle
Type c	Divisions above and below the undivided muscle
Type d	Undivided nerve between heads
Type e	Divisions between and above heads
Type f	Undivided nerve above the undivided muscle

Various researchers adopted this classification to categorize their findings. The two common groups of variations are the undivided sciatic nerve passing below the unsplit muscle. At the same time, the other is the unusual appearance of the sciatic nerve exiting the gluteal region and entering through the greater sciatic foramen as an early split into tibial and common peroneal nerves (Tomaszewski et al. 2016). There is a need to provide a compendious and evidence-based evaluation of composite anatomical variations of the sciatic nerve, piriformis muscle, and their relationship during routine dissection of cadavers.

2 Anatomy of the Piriformis Muscle and the Sciatic Nerve

The sciatic nerve is the largest nerve carrying ventral rami of L4-S3 spinal nerves, which lies inferior to the piriformis muscle in the gluteal region and is the longest and thickest nerve in the human body. It courses through the pelvis, passing beneath or through the piriformis muscle in approximately 85% of individuals. The provenance of the anatomical variation in the pelvic region is mostly embryologically influenced. The various sites of origin of the piriformis muscle include the second to fourth sacral segment (pelvic surface), the upper margin of the greater sciatic notch, and the sacrotuberous ligament. Post origin, it tends to exit the pelvis through the greater sciatic foramen along with the ischiadic nerve and inserts into the greater trochanter of the femur (Natsis et al. 2014; Parson 2009).

Its unique position and shape allow it to function as an external hip joint rotator, aiding in walking and running. The piriformis muscle and sciatic nerve are key players in the complex network of the human anatomy. This anatomical relationship poses a potential risk for compression or entrapment of the sciatic nerve by the piriformis muscle, leading to the development of piriformis syndrome (Berihu and Debeb 2015). In some individuals, the sciatic nerve may pass through the muscle belly itself, while in others, it may travel adjacent to or beneath it. This variability contributes to the complexity of diagnosing piriformis syndrome, as the same site and mechanism of nerve impingement may differ from person to person.

Muscular branches of the nerve are distributed to all the hamstrings. Sensory branches supply the whole tibial and foot areas except for the anteromedial tibial region and medial margin of the foot supplied by the saphenous nerve. The Tibial component is formed by a ventral branch of the ventral rami of L4 to S3 spinal nerves, while the dorsal branch of the ventral rami of L4 to S2 spinal nerves forms the common peroneal nerve. There is a high likelihood of variability of the sites of the division of the sciatic nerve into its components, where the commonest site is the junction of the middle and lower third of the thigh, near the popliteal fossa's apex (Amlan et al. 2023).

When the piriformis muscle becomes tight, inflamed, or hypertrophic, it can compress or irritate the sciatic nerve, resulting in a cascade of symptoms. The classic symptoms associated with piriformis syndrome include deep gluteal pain, radiating pain down the back of the thigh and leg, numbness, tingling, and even weakness in the affected limb. However, due to the shared pathways and overlapping symptoms with other conditions like lumbar disc herniation or spinal stenosis, accurately pinpointing the source of these symptoms becomes a diagnostic challenge. Therefore, understanding the intricate anatomy and relationship between the piriformis muscle and the sciatic nerve is crucial in unraveling the complexities of piriformis syndrome. By comprehending the potential sites of nerve entrapment and the mechanisms by which the piriformis muscle can impinge upon the sciatic nerve, healthcare professionals can navigate the diagnostic process more effectively and provide targeted treatment for those suffering from this enigmatic condition.

3 Diagnostic Challenges of Piriformis Syndrome

Piriformis syndrome presents a diagnostic challenge due to its complex nature and elusive symptoms. The condition involves dysfunction of the piriformis muscle, located deep in the gluteal region, which plays a crucial role in hip function. However, diagnosing piriformis syndrome proves difficult due to its overlap with sciatica, as the piriformis muscle and sciatic nerve are closely intertwined. The absence of definitive diagnostic tests, such as X-rays and MRIs, further complicates the process, as these imaging techniques may fail to capture the subtle changes in muscle morphology or detect nerve entrapment. As a result, patients often endure inconclusive examinations and trials, leading to uncertainty and frustration. Another challenge stems from the lack of universally accepted diagnostic criteria for piriformis syndrome. Clinicians rely on clinical signs, symptomatology, and physical examination findings to reach a diagnosis, but the subjective nature of pain, diverse symptom presentation, and overlap with other conditions often lead to misdiagnosis or delayed recognition. The complexity of piriformis syndrome is evident in its varied symptom manifestations. Some individuals experience localized buttock pain, while others endure radiating discomfort down the leg or numbness and tingling sensations. This diversity further complicates the identification and confirmation of the syndrome (Siddiq 2018; Chang et al. 2023).

4 Variations of the Piriformis Muscle, Sciatic Nerve and Piriformis Syndrome

Variations in the piriformis muscle, sciatic nerve, and the manifestations of piriformis syndrome further contribute to the diagnostic challenges associated with this condition. Anatomical variations of the piriformis muscle are not uncommon, with reports suggesting that the muscle may have different origins, insertions, or even absence in some individuals. These variations can alter the spatial relationship between the piriformis muscle and the sciatic nerve, potentially increasing the likelihood of nerve compression or entrapment.

Similarly, the sciatic nerve can exhibit variations in its course and relationship with the piriformis muscle. For example, in some individuals, the sciatic nerve may split into two distinct branches, passing either above or below the piriformis muscle. Alternatively, the nerve may have multiple divisions or communicate with other regional nerves. Such anatomical variations make it challenging to predict the precise location and mechanism of nerve compression, further complicating the diagnosis of piriformis syndrome.

Moreover, PS can manifest in diverse ways, with individual symptom presentation variations. For example, while the classic symptoms of deep gluteal pain and radiating leg pain are often reported, some patients may experience predominantly buttock pain without leg involvement. Others may present with symptoms mimicking lumbar radiculopathy, making it difficult to differentiate between piriformis syndrome and other conditions affecting the lower back and lower limb.

These variations in the piriformis muscle, sciatic nerve, and the clinical presentation of piriformis syndrome highlight the need for a comprehensive and individualized approach to diagnosis and management. Healthcare professionals must be aware of these anatomical variations and consider them when evaluating patients with suspected piriformis syndrome. In addition, a thorough history, physical examination, and diagnostic tests, such as electromyography and dynamic imaging, may be necessary to confirm the diagnosis and rule out other potential causes of similar symptoms.

In summary, the variations in the piriformis muscle, sciatic nerve, and the manifestations of piriformis syndrome contribute to the complexity of diagnosing this condition. Therefore, understanding and recognizing these variations is crucial for accurate diagnosis and effective treatment, ensuring that individuals suffering from piriformis syndrome receive the appropriate care tailored to their unique anatomical and symptomatic presentation.

5 Review of Literature

PS is considered an atypical, contentious neuromuscular disorder resulting from compression of the sciatic nerve at the level of the piriformis muscle. The diagnosis has been a major challenge due to difficulties finding the exact cause of the pain and a paucity of confirmed clinical and definitive diagnostic criteria like radio imaging or electrodiagnostic testing (Ro and Edmonds 2018; Miller et al. 2012). The anomalous variation of the sciatic nerve, piriformis muscle, and their variable relationship can lead to entrapment and nerve compression, resulting in piriformis syndrome (Adibatti and Sangeetha 2014). Such variations must be emphasized as they play a crucial role in the basis of sciatica and the pain etiology (Erdewyk 2017). Studies have explored various cadavers to provide awareness and strengthen the findings of the sciatic nerve variation and its relation to the piriformis as a probable cause for non-discogenic sciatica and other pain etiologies.

A study on 40 dissected gluteal regions in the Nepalese cadavers encountered 92.5% type-a, 2.5% type-b, and 5% type-c nerve-muscle relations (Jha and Baral 2020). This study also observed an altered anatomical variation where a higher sciatic nerve division occurs, and the common peroneal component passes between the two heads of the piriformis muscle (Fig. 1).

Another study from India revealed similar findings with 92% of type-a, 2% of type-b, and 6% of type-c with dissection on gluteal regions (Adibatti and Sangeetha 2014). Desalegn et al. found 92% of type-a, 3% of type-b, and 5.5% of type-c while dissecting 36 gluteal regions of the northern Ethiopian population (Desalegn and Tesfay 2014). Another study revealed 77% of type-a, 20% of type-b, and 3% of type-c from Polish cadavers (Haladaj et al. 2015). Berihu et al. research on 56 Ethiopian cadavers marked 89% of type-a, 9% of type-b and 2% of type-c relations (Berihu and Debeb 2015). Various studies on Turkish, Brazilian, and Kenyan cadavers reported 76%, 90%, and 90% type a relation and 24%, 10%, and 10% of type b-f relations, respectively (Guvencer et al. 2008; Brooks et al. 2011; Ogeng'o et al. 2011). Another substantial research resulted in 79% type-a, 14% type-b, 4% type-c, and 2% type-d relationship between the sciatic nerve and piriformis muscle in the Czech Republican cadavers (Pokorny et al. 2006). There was a similarity in a finding of research conducted on 100 Indian cadavers, which showed 85% type-a, 9% type-b, 3% type-c, and 3% type-d relations (Sinha et al. 2014). Studies have also revealed 2.2%, 10%, 0.35%, and 3% type-d relations, respectively (Natsis et al. 2014; Brooks et al. 2011; Pokorny et al. 2006; Sinha et al. 2014). Greek research on 290 cadavers revealed 0.35% extremely rare type-f relation (Natsis et al. 2014). Some studies on 24 Malaysian and 102 American cadavers have reported 83.4% and 88.2% type-a relations and 16.6% and 11.8% type b-f relations, respectively; however, type-d, type-e, and type-f relations were absent (Khan et al. 2016; Lewis et al. 2016). Another research on 120 American cadavers detected 97.5% type-a and 2.5% type-b relations (Erdewyk 2017).

Fetal cadaver research in the Turkish population revealed 98% type-a 1% type b, and 1% type c relations (Sulak et al. 2014). The probability of anatomical variation

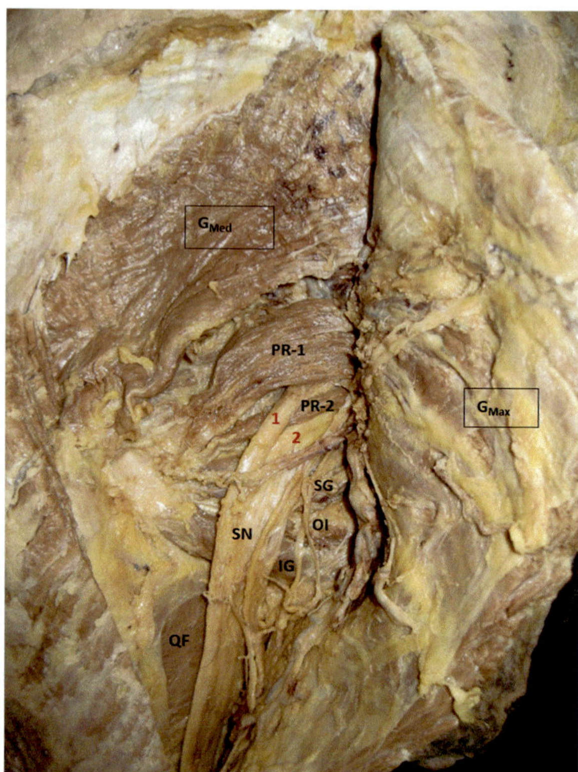

Fig. 1 Higher division of sciatic nerve and split piriformis muscle with two heads. 1: common peroneal superior head of piriformis; 2: tibial component; PR-1: inferior component; PR-2: head of piriformis; GMax: gluteus maximus; GMed: gluteus medius; SN: sciatic nerve; SG: superior gemellus. Figure from open access article: Original work: Jha AK, Baral P. Composite Anatomical Variations between the Sciatic Nerve and the Piriformis Muscle: A Nepalese Cadaveric Study. Case Rep Neurol Med. 2020 Mar 31;2020

in cadavers makes it essential for medical professionals to be aware of the potential complications during medical or surgical interventions (Smoll 2010). Jonathan et al. focused on the anatomical variation that plays a significant role in causing PS; however, the unassociated variations were ruled out due to the difficulty in their identification (Erdewyk 2017). The source of refractory sciatic pain due to anatomic variations is rare. Despite the recognition of these variations in the early twentieth century, these findings are uncommon both clinically and radiologically. This historical diagnostic difficulty arises due to the inability to localize the source of pain in PS. Therefore, it is usually a diagnosis of exclusion made by clinical findings (Cassidy et al. 2012).

Neuroimaging techniques are emerging and gaining popularity, and therefore, researchers and neuro physicians will benefit more precisely in recognizing, diagnosing, treating, and managing the pain associated with nerve entrapment due to composite piriformis-sciatic nerve anomalies. As a future implication, it is important to emphasize the study of the embryological basis of these structural variations and their origins.

Variations in the anatomical division of the sciatic nerve are commonly reported. An unusual variation of the sciatic nerve in relation to the superior gemellus and the presence of anomalous muscle has also been reported. The anomalous communicating branches of the posterior cutaneous femoral nerve with tibial and common peroneal nerve and the presence of an anomalous muscle originating from the greater sciatic notch and inserted at ischial tuberosity have been encountered during cadaveric dissections. A newer term, 'Sciaticotuberosus,' has been applied based on muscular attachments. Such variations hold clinical significance as they may contribute to piriformis syndrome, coccydynia, non-discogenic sciatica, and popliteal fossa block failure leading to local anesthesia toxicity and blood vessel traumatization (Amlan et al. 2023).

6 Conclusion

In this chapter, we have embarked on a journey into the intricate and perplexing world of piriformis syndrome, focusing on the composite anatomical variations between the sciatic nerve and the piriformis muscle that contribute to the diagnostic challenges associated with this condition. The piriformis muscle and the sciatic nerve, intimately intertwined within the gluteal region, have a delicate relationship that can become the root cause of piriformis syndrome. However, the complexity arises from the variations in their anatomical configuration, which significantly impact the likelihood and site of nerve impingement or compression.

Anatomical variations in the piriformis muscle can include differences in origin, insertion, or absence in some individuals. In addition, such variations alter the spatial relationship between the muscle and the sciatic nerve, creating a dynamic landscape where nerve compression may occur uniquely and unpredictably. These composite anatomical variations form the foundation of healthcare professionals' diagnostic challenges when differentiating piriformis syndrome from other conditions. The sciatic nerve itself is not exempt from variations. It can exhibit divergent courses and relationships with the piriformis muscle. For instance, the sciatic nerve may split into distinct branches, passing either above or below the piriformis muscle. Multiple divisions or communication with other nearby nerves can further complicate the situation. The resulting anatomical variations affect the mechanics of nerve impingement, making diagnosing piriformis syndrome a complex puzzle to solve.

When confronted with piriformis syndrome, clinicians must decipher this intricate interplay between the sciatic nerve and the piriformis muscle. The variability in their anatomy necessitates meticulously evaluating each patient's unique configuration, ensuring that no two cases are treated the same. In addition, it demands a comprehensive understanding of the variations and their potential impact on the manifestation of symptoms. Furthermore, the clinical presentation of piriformis syndrome varies from person to person, adding another layer of complexity. For example, some individuals may experience localized gluteal pain, while others may suffer from radiating pain down the leg or accompanying sensory disturbances. This diversity in symptomatology further emphasizes the significance of understanding the composite anatomical variations and their potential role in producing distinct patterns of pain and discomfort.

Despite the challenges posed by these composite anatomical variations, advances in diagnostic techniques offer hope for improved accuracy and efficiency. For example, dynamic imaging modalities, such as dynamic ultrasound, provide real-time visualization of the interaction between the piriformis muscle and the sciatic nerve, enabling healthcare professionals to identify abnormalities and better correlate them with clinical symptoms. These advancements pave the way for a more personalized and targeted approach to diagnosis and treatment.

In conclusion, the composite anatomical variations between the sciatic nerve and the piriformis muscle lie at the heart of the diagnostic challenges in piriformis syndrome. Understanding these variations and their impact on symptomatology is crucial for healthcare professionals striving to unravel the complexities of this condition. By embracing the nuances of anatomy, harnessing innovative diagnostic technologies, and tailoring treatment to individual presentations, we can navigate the intricate terrain of piriformis syndrome, ultimately providing relief and improved quality of life for those afflicted by this condition.

References

Adibatti M, Sangeetha V. Study on variant anatomy of sciatic nerve. J Clin Diagn Res. 2014;8(8):AC07–9.

Amlan A, Ansari AW, Bhingardeo AV, Chandrupatla M, Bojja S. A rare variation of high division of the sciatic nerve and associated neuromuscular variations in the Gluteal Region. Cureus. 2023;15(4): e37187.

Beaton LE, Anson BJ. The relation of the sciatic nerve and of its subdivisions to the piriformis muscle. Anat Rec. 1937;70(1):1–5.

Berihu BA, Debeb YG. Anatomical variation in bifurcation and trifurcations of sciatic nerve and its clinical implications: in selected university in Ethiopia. BMC Res Notes. 2015;8:633.

Brooks JBB, Silva CAC, Soares SA, Kai MR, Cabral RH, Fragoso YD. Variações anatômicas do nervo ciático em um grupo de cadáveres brasileiros. Revista Dor. 2011;12(4):332–6.

Cassidy L, Walters A, Bubb K, Shoja MM, Tubbs RS, Loukas M. Piriformis syndrome: implications of anatomical variations, diagnostic techniques, and treatment options. Surg Radiol Anat. 2012;34(6):479–86.

Chang A, Ly N, Varacallo M. Piriformis injection. StatPearls. Treasure Island (FL) 2023.

Erdewyk JIV. Anatomical variations of the sciatic nerve divisions in relation to the piriformis muscle and clinical implications [Theses & Dissertations]: University of Nebraska Medical Center; 2017.

Guvencer M, Akyer P, Iyem C, Tetik S, Naderi S. Anatomic considerations and the relationship between the piriformis muscle and the sciatic nerve. Surg Radiol Anat. 2008;30(6):467–74.

Haladaj R, Pingot M, Polguj M, Wysiadecki G, Topol M. Anthropometric study of the piriformis muscle and sciatic nerve: a morphological analysis in a Polish population. Med Sci Monit. 2015;21:3760–8.

Hicks BL, Lam JC, Varacallo M. Piriformis Syndrome. StatPearls. Treasure Island (FL) 2023.

Jha AK, Baral P. Composite anatomical variations between the sciatic nerve and the piriformis muscle: a Nepalese cadaveric study. Case Rep Neurol Med. 2020;2020:7165818.

Khan AA, Asari MA, Pasha MA. The sciatic nerve in human cadavers—high division or low formation? Folia Morphol (Warsz). 2016;75(3):306–10.

Lewis S, Jurak J, Lee C, Lewis R, Gest T. Anatomical variations of the sciatic nerve, in relation to the piriformis muscle. Transl Res Anat. 2016;5:15–9.

Desalegn M, Tesfay A. Variations of sciatic nerve its exit in relation to piriformis muscle in the Northern Ethiopia. Int J Pharma Sci Res. 2014;5(12):953–6.

Miller TA, White KP, Ross DC. The diagnosis and management of piriformis syndrome: myths and facts. Can J Neurol Sci. 2012;39(5):577–83.

Mitra SR, Roy S, Dutta AS, Ghosh A, Roy R, Jha AK. Piriformis syndrome: a review. J Evol Med Dent Sci. 2014;3:3804+.

Natsis K, Totlis T, Konstantinidis GA, Paraskevas G, Piagkou M, Koebke J. Anatomical variations between the sciatic nerve and the piriformis muscle: a contribution to surgical anatomy in piriformis syndrome. Surg Radiol Anat. 2014;36(3):273–80.

Ogeng'o JA, El-Busaidy H, Mwika PM, Khanbhai MM, Munguti J. Variant anatomy of sciatic nerve in a black Kenyan population. Folia Morphol (Warsz). 2011;70(3):175–9.

Parson SH. Clinically oriented anatomy, 6th edn. J Anat. 2009;215(4):474.

Pokorny D, Jahoda D, Veigl D, Pinskerova V, Sosna A. Topographic variations of the relationship of the sciatic nerve and the piriformis muscle and its relevance to palsy after total hip arthroplasty. Surg Radiol Anat. 2006;28(1):88–91.

Ro TH, Edmonds L. Diagnosis and management of piriformis syndrome: a rare anatomic variant analyzed by magnetic resonance imaging. J Clin Imaging Sci. 2018;8:6.

Siddiq MAB. Piriformis syndrome and wallet neuritis: are they the same? Cureus. 2018;10(5): e2606.

Sinha MB, Aggarwal A, Sahni D, Kaur H, Gupta R, Sinha HP. Morphological variations of sciatic nerve and piriformis muscle in gluteal region during fetal period. Eur J Anat. 2014;18:261–6.

Smoll NR. Variations of the piriformis and sciatic nerve with clinical consequence: a review. Clin Anat. 2010;23(1):8–17.

Sulak O, Sakalli B, Ozguner G, Kastamoni Y. Anatomical relation between sciatic nerve and piriformis muscle and its bifurcation level during fetal period in human. Surg Radiol Anat. 2014;36(3):265–72.

Tomaszewski KA, Graves MJ, Henry BM, Popieluszko P, Roy J, Pekala PA, et al. Surgical anatomy of the sciatic nerve: a meta-analysis. J Orthop Res. 2016;34(10):1820–7.

Yeoman W. The relation of Arthritis of the Sacro-Iliac joint to sciatica, with an analysis of 100 cases. The Lancet. 1928;212(5492):1119–23.

Piriformis Syndrome: Epidemiology, Clinical features, Diagnosis, and Treatment

Md. Abu Bakar Siddiq⊙, Israt Jahan, and Johannes J. Rasker

Abstract Piriformis syndrome (PS) is an example of extra-spinal sciatica that is often confused with spinal sciatica (prolapsed lumbar intervertebral disc), which makes diagnosis and treatment delay. The condition is not as rare as we believe; its prevalence is reported to vary between 0.3% and 36% among patients complaining of radiating low back pain. The female has a higher disease predilection; however, men also get the disease significantly. The most common complaint is a deep-seated gluteal pain that gets worse when sitting for a long time; walking usually intensifies the pain, but in chronic PS cases, ambulation may lessen pain. Moreover, Pace sign, FAIR (Flexion- Adduction-Internal Rotation of hip) test, Freiberg test, and Beatty tests are positive. Pain responds partially with analgesics and therapeutic exercise (stretching of piriformis muscle, PM), some may require ultrasound or fluoroscopy-guided steroid and botulinum toxin injections in PM. PS refractory to the above interventions may require surgery. PS is considered a chronic benign condition; however, deep-seated gluteal pain with raised ESR (Erythrocyte Sedimentation Rate), and CRP (C-Reactive Protein) because of piriformis pyomyositis as seen following vaginal delivery is an emergency and should be treated with judicial antibiotics and surgical drainage, where appropriate.

Md. Abu Bakar Siddiq (✉)
Department of Physical Medicine and Rehabilitation, Brahmanbaria Medical College, Brahmanbaria, Bangladesh
e-mail: abusiddiq37@yahoo.com

Department of Rheumatology, University of South Wales, Pontypridd, UK

I. Jahan
Department of Medical Biochemistry, Institute of Applied Health Science, [IAHS], Chittagong, Bangladesh

J. J. Rasker
Department of Psychology Health and Technology, Faculty of Behavioural Sciences, University of Twente, Enschede, The Netherlands

Md. Abu Bakar Siddiq
Department of Rheumatology, Faculty of Medicine and Health Science, Kolling Institute, Royal North Shore Hospital, University of Sydney, Sydney, Australia

                    75
K. M. Iyer (ed.), *Piriformis Syndrome*,
https://doi.org/10.1007/978-3-031-40736-9_15

Keywords Piriformis muscle · Piriformis syndrome · Epidemiology · Clinical features · Diagnosis · Treatment

Key Messages

- Piriformis syndrome is an example of extra-spinal sciatica
- Piriformis syndrome is a disorder of exclusion of its mimics
- The simultaneous presence of Spinal sciatica (prolapsed lumbar intervertebral disc) and extra-spinal sciatica, for example PS, could result in further diagnostic delay
- Piriformis syndrome is generally benign and more often seen in women
- Piriformis pyomyositis or PS due to cervical cancer may mistakenly be diagnosed and treated as piriformis syndrome.

1 Introduction

Piriformis Syndrome (PS) is an example of extra-spinal sciatica and has also been described as 'deep gluteal syndrome', 'pelvic outlet syndrome' or 'pseudo-sciatica'. PS is characterized by localized gluteal and radiating low back pain (LBP) caused by a spasmodic piriformis muscle (PM) and compressed, irritated and stretched sciatic nerve (SN) behind the PM (Siddiq et al. 2017). Physicians may consider it an orthopedic condition, some categorize it as a neurological disorder, whereas others classify it as a soft-tissue rheumatism of the PM (Siddiq et al. 2020). The Greek doctor Hippocrates (460–370 BC) already used the *term* 'sciatica' or ischias (Greek ἰσχιάς)) for pain irradiating from the os ischii down the leg (Stafford et al. 2007). In the nineteenth century, Lasègue described a provocative test for sciatica pain of disc disorders (Stafford et al. 2007). Later, Mixter and Barr described how intervertebral disc prolapse compressing adjacent SN roots generate sciatica-like pain (Mixter and Barr 1934). Pain in lumbago sciatica is the result of an inflammatory response of the SN to prolapsed disc materials, whereas nerve root compression contributes to functional impairment. In some cases, PS may mimic prolapsed lumbar intervertebral disc (PLID), hence being misdiagnosed and wrongly treated without significant relief. The simultaneous presence of lumbago sciatica and extra-spinal sciatica, for example PS, could result in further diagnostic delay (Siddiq et al. 2020). In this chapter, we focus on anatomy of piriformis muscle and nerve, epidemiology, clinical features, differential diagnosis and treatment of PS.

2   Anatomy of Piriformis Muscle and Nerve

The Musculus (M) piriformis is a flat, pear-shaped muscle located in the gluteal region and proximal thigh (Fig. 1). It courses underneath the gluteus maximus, parallel to the posterior margin of the gluteus medius. The PM originates mainly from the anterior surface of the lateral process of the sacrum, the spinal region of the gluteal muscles, and the gluteal surface of the ilium close to the greater sciatic notch, the capsule of sacroiliac joint, and the sacrotuberous ligament (Chang et al. 2022). The muscle passes through the greater sciatic notch dividing it into superior and inferior compartments and inserts on the medial aspect of the superior greater trochanter of the femur. Before inserting into the femur, the PM tendon forms a conjoint tendon with other hip abductors. The sciatic nerve, leaves the pelvis through the greater sciatic notch remaining behind the PM; however, clinically important congenital anomalies of PM have been described in relation to PS (Chang et al. 2022; Boyajian-O'Neil et al. 2008) (Fig. 1a, b). The PM is an external rotator of the hip during the hip extension and abducts the femur during flexion of the hip. The hip abduction while walking shifts body weight and protect us from falling. The PM receives innervation from L5, S1, and S2 nerves and important in keeping PM functional.

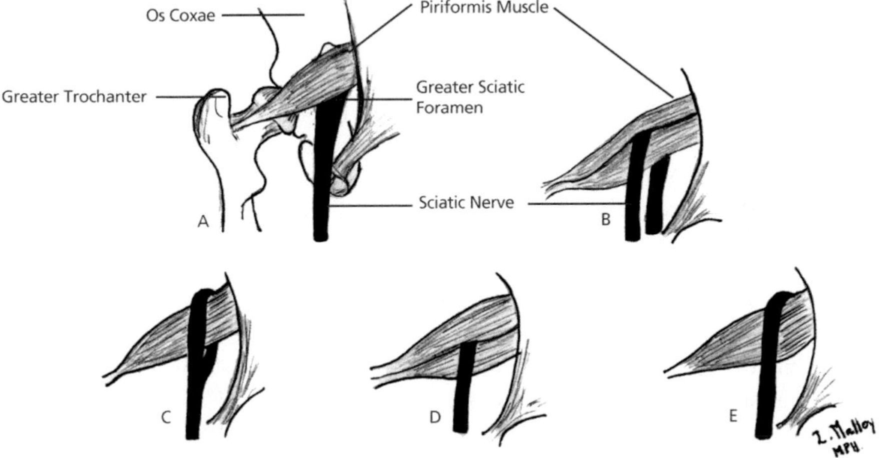

Fig. 1 a Anatomy of hip rotators including piriformis muscle and sciatic nerve in relation to piriformis syndrome (Boyajian-O'Neil et al. 2008; Hopayian et al. 2010); b, variations in relationship of the sciatic nerve to the piriformis muscle (all deep gluteal muscles have been removed, PM has been shown from back): (A) the sciatic nerve exiting the greater sciatic foramen along the inferior surface of the piriformis muscle; the sciatic nerve splitting as it passes through the piriformis muscle with the tibial branch passing (B) Anatomy of hip rotators including piriformis muscle and sciatic nerve in relation to piriformis syndrome

3 Pathophysiology of Piriformis Syndrome

When the PM is overused and/or inflamed, it irritates the adjacent SN with clinical features characteristic of lumbago sciatica. Isolated PM spasm due to chronic poor body posture or some acute injury resulting in a sudden and strong internal rotation of the hip may lead to PS (Hicks et al. 2022). After a fall or direct gluteal blow, a localized hematoma may heal with scar formation in the area between the sciatic nerve and hip extensor, including PM. Sometimes, altered biomechanics of spine and gluteal structures in patients with leg length discrepancy (LLD) may lead to ipsilateral or bilateral PS development (Gerwin 2001).

Extreme use of the PM during long-distance walking, running, repeated squatting, rowing/sculling, kneeling, bicycling, etc. also may result in PS. In some patients PS may be due to myofascial pain syndrome (MPS) involving the PM with taut bands and painful, tender trigger points (TrPs) (Gerwin 2001). Although MPS is a localized painful muscle condition, sometimes it may be widespread due to spreading TrPs from PM to adjacent axial muscle chain of back (Gerwin 2001). Widespread MPS sometimes may get confused with generalized body ache as seen in FMS, an example of central sensitization; sometimes, both conditions may co-exist in the same patient and share a common pathophysiology. MPS patients may have one or more episodes a profound form before they develop FMS (Gerwin 2001). In MPS-PM, an increase in TrPs acetylcholine release at the neuromuscular junction may lead to sustained depolarization of the post-junctional membrane of the muscle fibre producing sarcomere contraction with increased local energy consumption and compromised circulation with resultant hypoxia to PM (Gerwin 2001). The localized muscle ischemia leads to release of substance P that sensitizes PM and afferent nerve nociceptors in the dorsal horn and spinal neurons with pain referral beyond the initial nociceptive region (Siddiq et al. 2017). Thus MPS in PM may contribute to developing widespread body ache (Siddiq et al. 2017; Siddiq et al. 2020; Gerwin 2001).

PS is an example of pseudo-sciatica, thus, before planning an intervention in a patient with sciatica, it is of paramount importance to differentiate between spinal sciatica and extra-spinal pseudo-sciatica (Siddiq et al. 2020). PS in association with lumbar spinal stenosis has also been described, being explained by the "double crush hypothesis" (axons compressed at one site could also get compressed at another site) as explained by Upton and McComas in 1973 (Siddiq and Rasker 2018). Anatomical variations of PM may contribute to PS manifestations (Boyajian-O'Neil et al. 2008) (Fig. 1b).

4   Epidemiology – prevalence and risk factors (occupations, sex distribution, and seasonal variations)

According to various reports, PS may be responsible for between 0.33 and 36% of all causes of low back pain and or sciatica. (Siddiq et al. 2017). It is common in middle-aged people (mean age 38 years) with a predominance among women; however, men also can get the disorder (Siddiq et al. 2017). A wide Q-angle in women may contribute to PS; if this is the case, PS could be bilateral but till date no medical report described bilateral PS in women. In our previous study different occupations have been found to be associated with PS; however, due to the small sample size we could not analyze whether occupation has any significant causal link with PS or whether they differ depending on the gender (Siddiq et al. 2017). Increased PM thickness in PS as measured by high-frequency musculoskeletal ultrasonography (MSUS) has been reported in a cross-sectional analytic study by Siahaan et al. (1.16 ± 0.13 versus 0.85 ± 0.11 cm, respectively for the PS and healthy side, $p < 0.05$) (Siahaan et al. 2021). However, inconsistent clinical features and clinical mimics of PS from surrounding gluteal structures may vary in different geographical areas, cultures, and socioeconomic conditions. As demonstrated in our recent article, the demographic data of PS patients depicted average age at presentation was 43 years, and all patients were within the 21–60 age group (Siddiq et al. 2017). Women had more PS than men (Siddiq et al. 2017). More PS among homemakers and more patients were from rural areas. However, these demographic data may differ if a large study sample is included.

There are *primary and secondary* forms of PS. In primary PS, there is spasm and hypertrophy of the piriformis muscle (PM) without any recognizable cause, sometimes it may be due to anomalous sciatic nerve and PM (Fig. 1b). Secondary PS may happen in patients with lumbar spinal canal stenosis, MPS of PM, long-distance walking, due to occupations (e.g. dancing), myositis ossificans of PM, leg length discrepancy (LLD), etc. (Siddiq et al. 2017; Siddiq et al. 2017). Sometimes, usage of fatty back wallet (walletosis) in men may induce PS (Siddiq et al. 2017).

PS may be seen in women with fibromyalgia (FMS) (Siddiq et al. 2014). PS has also been described in women with iron-deficiency anemia (IDA) and rheumatoid arthritis (RA), improving with blood transfusion and non-steroidal anti-inflammatory drugs (NSAIDs) respectively (Siddiq et al. 2017).

Many patients suggest that the weather may influence their LBP and some associations have been confirmed in several studies Temperature and humidity influence chronic or recurrent self-reported LBP. In a study in England, chronic widespread pain sufferers had most pain in winter, intermediate in autumn and spring, and lowest in summer. However, further research is needed to explore any association between the incidence of acute LBP with precipitation, humidity, wind speed, gust, and direction, and air pressure (Siddiq et al. 2023). PS is a rare type of LBP. The correlation between PS incidence and season changes has never been studied. In a pilot study, we studied whether the pattern of PS, the frequency of PS were associated with PS manifestations over two different seasons (Siddiq et al. 2023). PS was seen more during dry winter and pre-monsoon, and less in rainy monsoon; however, further research with large number of patients are needed. (Siddiq et al. 2023).

Walletosis, or fat-wallet syndrome, or credit-card neuritis have synonymously but incorrectly been used for deep gluteal PS (Siddiq et al. 2017; Siddiq 2018). In 1966, the first case of wallet neuritis was published. Sometimes, the long-standing use of fatty wallets loaded with unnecessary scraps (even without credit-card), like papers, visiting cards, etc., could result in features resembling SN neuritis (Siddiq et al. 2017). Later, in 1978, Lutz reported two cases of credit-card-wallet sciatica with even a small-sized wallet (Lutz 1978). In our recent case series, we described wallet neuritis in three different professionals (a doctor, a banker, and a day laborer), improving with mere discontinuation of using a buttock wallet, wallectomy! (Siddiq et al. 2017; Siddiq 2018).

Cervical cancer in women may spread to gluteal muscles, including PM resulting in PS, and also radiotherapy for cervical malignancy may cause atrophy of PM inducing or mimicking PS (Siddiq and Rasker 2018). In our recent systematic review, we depicted how purulent PM myositis may develop in women following vaginal delivery and also after abortion, resulting in a medical emergency; these patients usually report deep-seated persistent gluteal pain, fever, and raised inflammatory markers (Siddiq and Rasker 2019). We describe this condition below in more detail.

5 Diagnosis of Piriformis Syndrome

PS is a disorder of diagnostic exclusion of its mimics. Usually, PS presents with localized buttock and deep-seated gluteal pain with variable irradiation and intensity and typical pain aggravating and relieving factors. The pain aggravates with sitting longer, and walking relieves pain, especially in chronic cases (Siddiq et al. 2017). In acute conditions, differentiating PS from PLID is really tough, a situation when PS could be over-diagnosed or underdiagnosed. Immediate clinical differentiation between them can be difficult and MRI of the lumbosacral spine often needed for diagnosis. A positive SLR raising test favors lumbar nerve root compression in PLID; however, in acute PS, patients may also have difficulty in raising the ipsilateral leg and this finding may cause further diagnostic delay. In our recent study, we described PS features in 31 patients (male: female = 1:2) (Siddiq et al. 2017): buttock pain was seen in all patients; pain was aggravated with long-time sitting and affected side-lying. Pain also aggravated during standing from sitting (77.4%), and forward bending (90.3%). Besides, associated tingling feeling according to sciatic nerve distribution was reported in 90.3% cases, 19.35% reported considerable pain improvement while walking. Gluteal tenderness, positive FAIR test, and the Pace sign were elicited in all patients (Siddiq et al. 2017). Palpable gluteal mass and gluteal atrophy was documented in few of them. Straight leg raising test was positive in acute PS cases. High-frequency diagnostic MSUS depicted increased PM thickness on the affected side (Siddiq et al. 2017). There are no diagnostic criteria set for the disorder. In a recent systematic review, Hopayian et al. described the following common features in PS:

buttock pain with external tenderness over the greater sciatic notch, and gluteal pain aggravated through sitting are common. Maneuvers like flexion-adduction-internal rotation (FAIR) test, the Pace sign, the Freiberg test, and digital rectal examination are useful in defining PS (Hopayian et al. 2010). PS is of primary and secondary. In our recent study, we depicted secondary PS and PS-like features in association with preceding fall, rheumatoid arthritis, overuse of PM, lumbar spinal stenosis, FMS, intra-muscular gluteal injection, blunt buttock trauma, leg length discrepancy (LLD), and use of rear pocket's wallet (Siddiq et al. 2017).

Table 1 lists clinical maneuvers that are useful in PS diagnosis. External gluteal tenderness with 'sausage mass' of PM spasm in an area between the greater sciatic notch and the greater trochanter is common (Boyajian-O'Neil et al. 2008). The FAIR test is the most sensitive test and is used widely to diagnose PS (Boyajian-O'Neil et al. 2008). The test is performed in supine position, keeping affected hip flexed at 60° and knee flexed at 90° followed by internal rotation and adduction of the hip joint (Hopayian et al. 2010). In a modified FAIR test, the FAIR test is done in combination with Lasègue's sign, as described by Chen et al. (Chen and Nizar 2013). The Pace sign (resisted abduction and external rotation of the thigh) is reported to be positive in 30–74% (Hopayian et al. 2010). The Pace manoeuver induces gluteal pain on resisted abduction of the flexed hip while sitting (Siddiq et al. 2017; Hopayian et al. 2010). The Freiberg sign (forceful internal rotation of the extended thigh) and the Pace sign are found to be positive, respectively, in 56.2 and 46.5% of the PS patients (Siddiq et al. 2017). The medial end of the PM can be palpated within the pelvis by rectal or vaginal examination, and this test is positive in almost 100% of the patients (Siddiq et al. 2017). Digital rectal examination is the most commonly used internal pain provocation technique for PS, and the finding was considered to be positive provided that patients did jump or changed facial expression during finger gliding over the lateral pelvic wall (Siddiq et al. 2017; Hopayian et al. 2010). The Beatty test is also useful in PS diagnosis.

Besides clinical features, radio-imaging help PS diagnosis. MSUS-guided lidocaine (2%) injection in PM relieving gluteal pain may be both diagnostic and therapeutic (Siddiq et al. 2017). MSUS (PM increased thickness), MRI (hypertrophy of PM), and NCS (nerve conduction study)/electromyogram (EMG) (suggest delayed response when is hip held in FAIR position) are useful in delineating deep-seated gluteal structures and excluding PS mimics (Siddiq et al. 2017; Siahaan et al. 2021). The electrophysiologic approach has been used to diagnose PS by noting the presence of H waves (Siddiq et al. 2017; Hopayian et al. 2010). MRI neurography may show the presence of irritation of the sciatic nerve just adjacent to the sciatic notch; however, it is not readily available in all clinics (Hopayian et al. 2010; Misirlioglu et al. 2018). Sometimes, surgical exploration of the PM may reveal PM calcification, SN impingement between hip abductors, anomalous PM and SN (Hopayian et al. 2010; Foster 2002; Beauchesne and Schutzer 1997).

Table 1 Clinical maneuvers are useful in piriformis syndrome diagnosis (Siddiq et al. 2017; Hopayian et al. 2010)

Name	Description
Lase'gue sign	Localized pain elicited if pressure is applied directly over the piriformis muscle and its tendon, especially with 90° hip flexion and extended knee
Freiberg test	Gluteal pain is experienced during the passive internal rotation of the extended hip
Pace sign	Resisted hip abduction when patients remained seated with flexed knees
Piriformis sign	Gluteal pain with externally rotated ipsilateral foot, a positive piriformis sign
FAIR	Hip flexion, adduction and internal rotation reproduces gluteal pain
Beatty	Patient lying on the asymptomatic side with flexed hip and knee reproduces pain with thigh abduction against gravity
Palpable gluteal mass	Palpable *'sausage-shaped'* mass in the buttock, an evidence of the piriformis muscle spasm
Per-rectal examination	Positive digital rectal examination signifies patients jump or change facial expression during finger gliding over the lateral pelvic wall on digital rectal examination
Diagnostic block	MSUS-guided diagnostic block of the nerve supplying piriformis muscle can be performed at 1.5 cm lateral and 1.2 cm caudal to the lower 1/3rd of the sacroiliac joint with 5 ml of 1% lignocaine injection. If pain is reduced, then the test is regarded positive

FAIR flexion, abduction and internal rotation of the hip

6 Differential Diagnosis

PS is a disorder of exclusion. Sometimes, PS diagnosis is not straightforward, and it may become a diagnostic difficulty. In a recent scoping review article, we described conditions mimicking PS (Table 2) (Siddiq et al. 2020).

7 Piriformis Syndrome-Like Presentation in Emergency

PS is not always benign. Sometimes, an infected PM leads to pyomyositis and deserves special attention. Skeletal pyomyositis follows three distinct phases—invasive stage (myositis without abscess formation), suppurative stage (myositis with abscess formation), and late stage with sepsis (consistent fever, septicemia, toxic and/ or coma) that requires intensive management). Staphylococcus aureus is the most common pathogen; however, Group A, as well as Group β Streptococcus, Salmonella typhi, Proteus mirabilis, Brucella melitensis, and *Escherichia coli*, also contribute to the pathogenesis (Siddiq 2018).

Table 2 Conditions mimicking piriformis syndrome (Siddiq et al. 2017; 2020; Hopayian et al. 2010)

Clinical conditions	Description
Wallet neuritis	Walletosis or Fat-wallet neuritis can mimics PS features. Discontinuation of wallet could improve the condition
Piriformis pyomyositis	Persistent deep-seated gluteal pain with fever, raised inflammatory markers positive PS maneuvers, MRI and MSUS-based space occupying lesion in PM is suggestive of piriformis pyomyositis. Common pathogens are—*Staphylococcus aureus, Group A Streptococci, Escherichia coli, Proteus Mirabilis, and Brucella Melitensis*
Superior cluneal nerve (SCN) disorder	LBP and leg pain are aggravated by standing, walking, bending from the waist, twisting, stairs up-down, and lifting weights. Tenderness over the posterior superior iliac crest reproduces the pain. In older people, SCN may be associated with a dorso-lumbar vertebral fracture
Quadratus lumborum (QL) and Gluteal medius myofascial pain syndrome (MPS)	QL trigger points (TPs) refer to pain in the SI joint, lower buttock and lateral hip regions and have the potential to generate distant TPs in gluteus muscles. Gluteal medius tendinitis (GMT) may also present with gluteal pain with pain referral to the thigh back, limited range-of-motion of the hip joint, fever, and raised inflammatory biomarkers that could mimic PS
Osteitis condensans illi (OCI) and SpA	OCI is seen in young women of childbearing age. LBP with pain referral to the thigh back is the presenting complaint. Pain aggravates with sitting and forward bending; however, lying relieves pain. X-ray sacroiliac joint reveals radio-opaque sclerotic change involving the ilial part of the SI joint, though sparing the SI joint. In SpA, inflammatory spinal pain is the presenting feature. Patients may be positive for HLA-B27 with high inflammatory biomarkers
Catamenial sciatica	According to the sciatic nerve distribution, radiating gluteal pain appears cyclically with menstruation and is sometimes associated with lower limb weakness, muscle wasting, reduced jerks, and impaired sensation. Advanced imaging with MRI and CT scan of the lumbosacral spine/pelvis and ultrasonogram of the whole abdomen help diagnose the condition. NCV/EMG demonstrates nerve damage
Post-injection sciatica	Sciatic nerve (SN) injury with sciatica-like features mimicking PS may develop following IM gluteal injection (more with NSAID, penicillin G, and diazepam). Clinical manifestations include sensory disturbance and foot drop with deformity (equinovarus, calcaneocavus or equinus)

(continued)

Table 2 (continued)

Clinical conditions	Description
Sciatic nerve sheath tumor	SN sheath tumor, for example, schwannoma, may present with sciatica-like features. MRI, US scanning of SN, and histopathology findings may help diagnose the lesion and exclude the differential diagnosis
Compressive neuropathy	The lateral cutaneous nerve of the thigh (LCNT), saphenous, sural, and common peroneal nerve compression could mimic lumbago. Lipoma, schwannoma, and ganglion cysts could compress SN at different levels. MSUS and MRI help diagnose them

FAIR flexion-adduction-internal rotation, *PR* per-rectal, *IL* intra-lesional, *NSAID* non-steroidal anti-inflammatory drug, PM: piriformis muscle, *SN* sciatic nerve, *MRI* magnetic resonance imaging, *MSUS* musculoskeletal ultrasound, *LBP* low back pain, *SI* sacroiliac, *CT* computed tomography, PRP: platelet rich plasma, SpA: spondyloarthropathy, *NCV* nerve conduction velocity, *EMG* electromyogram, *IM* intramuscular

Piriformis pyomyositis can develop in women after abortion and following vaginal, forceps, and ventouse delivery. Patients might get PM infection through transient bacteremia from intravenous cannula-associated cellulitis or seeding of infectious agents into PM might happen through the torn vaginal structures. Patients may have bacterial growth (Group β-streptococcus) in blood culture, some may have high vaginal swab growth of *Escherichia coli*, moderate growth of Group βstreptococcus, and mixed anaerobes. Besides, mixed growth could be found in mid-stream urine. Sometimes, an MRI of the pelvis revealed a high signal intensity signifies edematous and swollen PM compatible with purulent myositis with deep-seated gluteal pain and sciatica-like complaints. Purulent PS in type 2 diabetic women has also been reported (Siddiq 2018).

Piriformis pyomyositis in association with septic arthritis of the sacroiliac joint has been reported in children: patients reported high-grade fever, pin-point gluteal pain, and MRI-depicted space-occupying lesion involving greater sciatic notch and lumbar nerve roots. In adolescents hip pain due to piriformis pyomyositis may be reported at the emergency with positive SLR, fever with rigor, and sweating; later pelvic MRI T1-weighted imaging could reveal abnormally high signal intensity in PM, gadolinium administration could reveal the widespread extension of the lesion to soft tissue. Besides, the agglutination test could yield high titre for Brucella melitensis, and blood culture yields Brucella melitensis growth (Siddiq 2018).

Piriformis pyomyositis in men with gluteal pain and positive blood and or pus culture for Salmonella typhi. Apparently healthy tennis and rugby players could present with gluteal pain and MRI could depict fluid accumulation in the left iliopsoas, sacroiliac joint, and an SOL within the PM, patients had raised inflammatory biomarkers and blood cultures were positive for Staphylococcus aureus. In competitive swimmers, Proteus mirabilis-induced piriformis pyomyositis has also been reported. MRI/CT abdomen and pelvis revealed PM swelling. Patients also had raised ESR, CRP, and leukocytosis. Piriformis pyomyositis complicated with an extensive epidural abscess had also been reported, and culture from pus could yield methicillin-sensitive Staphylococcus aureus (Siddiq 2018).

Antibiotic treatment is the mainstay of piriformis pyomyositis treatment. Besides, patients may require NSAIDs, analgesics, and sedatives. The duration of antibiotic treatment may vary, and depends on the culprit organism types; however, initial intravenous regimen followed by oral therapy for a total of 3–8 weeks is well practiced. No intra-lesional (IL) corticosteroid or botox should be given. CT-guided aspiration followed by culture and sensitivity (C/S) test helps to confirm the diagnosis. Sometimes, no causative agent could be found. Start treatment with broad-spectrum antibiotic, then change it according to pus and blood C/S report. Empirical oral antibiotic therapy for example, oral Cefdinir (10 mg/kg/day) is found effective in pediatric patients. Empirical intravenous cloxacillin (1000 mg 8-hourly) or augmentin (1.2 g every 8 hours) or cefuroxime (750 mg, 3 times/day) followed by their oral formulations also improved pyomyositis in staphylococcus aureus sensitive cases. IV cloxacillin (2 weeks) and amikacin, oral cloxacillin are effective in methicilin-resistant Staphylococcus aureus. Intravenous vancomycin and meropenem are effective where cloxacillin becomes failed in Staphylococcus aureus-positive cases (Siddiq 2018).

Brucellosis also contributes in purulent piriformis myositis and combined doxycycline (100 mg 2 times/day), rifampin 900 mg (once/day), and ciprofloxacin (500 mg 2 times/day) regime relieves from brucellosis myositis. Intravenous vancomycin—15 mg/kg/12-hourly), followed by oral therapy (160 mg trimethoprim/800 mg sulfamethoxazole every 12 h), benzylpenicillin and clindamycin secures overall improvement in Group β-streptococcus and *E. coli* sensitive pyomyositis. Cefotaxime and tobramycin are found effective in Proteus Mirabilis (Siddiq 2018).

8   Treatment of Piriformis Syndrome

Short-term rest can relieve symptoms. Besides, soft tissue mobilizing can be beneficial. Non-steroidal anti-inflammatory drugs (NSAIDs) such as ibuprofen may alleviate the symptoms and provide short-term pain relief. Neuropathic agents such as gabapentin and pregabalin can be adjuncts to NSAIDs. The role of vitamin B preparations in PS treatment is inconclusive. Traditional stretching of gluteal musculatures and pulsed radiofrequency help some patients. Acupuncture shows some promise in the disorder. In some patients, MSUS-guided dry needling may be useful (Vij et al. 2021; Payne 2016).

MSUS-guided injection of lidocaine (2%) and betamethasone in the PM may produce statistically significant pain relief though for short-term periods, and repeated injection may be required (Payne 2016). There is no statistically significant difference between fluoroscopy and ultrasound-guided PM interventions. Some patients may find SN peri-neural corticosteroid injection effective. Injection of botulinum toxin type A (100–200 unit of BoNT-A) inhibiting the release of substance

P at the NMJ of PM could be useful in PS; however, Botox should be preserved for those who do not improve with other interventions (Vij et al. 2021; Fritz et al. 2014).

Surgical management of PS involves dissection of PM and decompression of the SN and can be done open or endoscopically; however, the endoscopic approach has some superiority in terms of improved visualization of PM muscle, less soft-tissue damage and postoperative pain, and reduced recovery times (Vij et al. 2021; Kay et al. 2017).

In summary, piriformis syndrome is an example of extra-spinal sciatica and a disorder of exclusion of many causes of low back pain. A logical diagnostic approach and imaging may make diagnosis of piriformis syndrome possible and should be followed to exclude PS mimics clinically. Pain killers may cause temporary pain relief; however, some patients need guided intervention, and some may benefit from surgery. Purulent piriformis myositis with PS-like deep-seated gluteal pain develop following vaginal delivery with fever, persistent gluteal pain, and raised inflammatory markers could be misdiagnosed as PS and corticosteroid injection in piriformis muscle may cause harm, while these patients need antibiotic therapy. So, PS is not always benign, sometimes it may even be an emergency.

References

Beauchesne RP, Schutzer SF. Myositis ossificans of the piriformis muscle: an unusual cause of piriformis syndrome. A case report. J Bone Joint Surg. 1997;79:906–910.

Boyajian-O'Neil LA, McClain RL, Coleman MK, Thomas PP. Diagnosis and management of piriformis syndrome: an osteopathic approach. J Am Osteopath Assoc. 2008;108:657–64.

Chang C, Jeno SH, Varacallo M. Anatomy, Bony Pelvis and lower limb: piriformis muscle. Updated 2022 Oct 3. In: StatPearls (Internet). Treasure Island (FL): StatPearls Publishing; 2023. Available from: https://www.ncbi.nlm.nih.gov/books/NBK519497/

Chen CK, Nizar AJ. Prevalence of piriformis syndrome in chronic low back pain patients. A clinical diagnosis with modified FAIR test. Pain Pract. 2013;13:276–281 J 19:2095–2101.

Foster MR. Piriformis syndrome. Orthopedics. 2002;25:821–5.

Fritz J, Chhabra A, Wang KC, Carrino JA. Magnetic resonance neurography-guided nerve blocks for the diagnosis and treatment of chronic pelvic pain syndrome. Neuroimaging Clin N Am. 2014;24(1):211–34. https://doi.org/10.1016/j.nic.2013.03.028.

Gerwin RD. Classification, epidemiology, and natural history of myofascial pain syndrome. Curr Pain Headache Rep. 2001;5:412–20.

Hicks BL, Lam JC, Varacallo M. Piriformis syndrome. Updated 2022 Sep 4. In: StatPearls (Internet). Treasure Island (FL): StatPearls Publishing; 2023. Available from: https://www.ncbi.nlm.nih.gov/books/NBK448172/

Hopayian K, Song F, Riera R, Sambandan S. The clinical features of the piriformis syndrome: a systemic review. Eur Spine J. 2010;19:2095–101.

Kay J, de Sa D, Morrison L, Fejtek E, Simunovic N, Martin HD, et al. Surgical management of deep gluteal syndrome causing sciatic nerve entrapment: a systematic review. Arthroscopy. 2017;33(12):2263–2278 e1. https://doi.org/10.1016/j.arthro.2017.06.041.

Lutz EG. Credit-card-wallet sciatica. JAMA. 1978;240(8):738 PMID: 671698.

Misirlioglu TO, Palamar D, Akgun K. Letter to the editor involving the article 'piriformis muscle syndrome: a cross-sectional imaging study in 116 patients and evaluation of therapeutic outcome.' Eur Radiol. 2018;28(12):5354–5.

Mixter WJ, Barr JS. Rupture of the intervertebral disc with involvement of the spinal canal. N Engl J Med. 1934;211:210–5.

Payne JM. Ultrasound-Guided hip procedures. Phys Med Rehabil Clin N Am. 2016;27(3):607–29. https://doi.org/10.1016/j.pmr.2016.04.004.

Siahaan YMT, Tiffani P, Tanasia A. Ultrasound-Guided measurement of piriformis muscle thickness to diagnose piriformis syndrome. Front Neurol. 2021;7(12):721966. https://doi.org/10.3389/fneur.2021.721966.

Siddiq MAB. Piriformis syndrome and wallet neuritis: are they the same? Cureus. 2018;10(5):e2606. https://doi.org/10.7759/cureus.2606.

Siddiq AB, Rasker JJ. Piriformis syndrome: still unsolved issues. Int J Clin Rheumatol. 2018;13(6):338–40.

Siddiq MAB, Rasker JJ. Piriformis pyomyositis, a cause of piriformis syndrome-a systematic search and review. Clin Rheumatol. 2019;38(7):1811–21. https://doi.org/10.1007/s10067-019-04552-y.(12).

Siddiq MA, Khasru MR, Rasker JJ. Piriformis syndrome in fibromyalgia: clinical diagnosis and successful treatment. Case Rep Rheumatol. 2014;2014:893836. https://doi.org/10.1155/2014/893836.

Siddiq MA, Hossain MS, Uddin MM, Jahan I, Khasru MR, Haider NM, Rasker JJ. Piriformis syndrome: a case series of 31 Bangladeshi people with literature review. Eur J Orthop Surg Traumatol. 2017;27(2):193–203. https://doi.org/10.1007/s00590-016-1853-0.

Siddiq MAB, Clegg D, Hasan SA, Rasker JJ. Extra-spinal sciatica and sciatica mimics: a scoping review. Korean J Pain. 2020;33(4):305–17. https://doi.org/10.3344/kjp.2020.33.4.305.

Siddiq MAB, Hossain MS, Khan AUA, Sayed MA, Rasker JJ. Piriformis syndrome in pre-monsoon, monsoon, and winter: an observational pilot study. Cureus. 2023;15(2):e35296. https://doi.org/10.7759/cureus.35296.

Siddiq AB, Jahan I, Alpha M. Wallet neuritis—an example of peripheral sensitization. Curr Rheum Rev. 2017;13(999). https://doi.org/10.2174/1573397113666170310100851.

Stafford MA, Peng P, Hill DA. Sciatica: a review of history, epidemiology, pathogenesis, and the role of epidural steroid injection in management. Br J Anaesth. 2007;99:461–73.

Vij N, Kiernan H, Bisht R, Singleton I, Cornett EM, Kaye AD, Imani F, Varrassi G, Pourbahri M, Viswanath O, Urits I. Surgical and non-surgical treatment options for piriformis syndrome: a literature review. Anesth Pain Med. 2021;11(1):e112825. https://doi.org/10.5812/aapm.112825.

Peroneal Neuropathy in Piriformis Syndrome

Gamze Gül Güleç

1   Introduction

Piriformis syndrome (PS) is a neuromuscular disorder that occurs when the piriformis muscle compresses or irritates the sciatic nerve or other anatomical structures that pass under the piriformis muscle (Kirschner et al. 2009). This compression can cause a range of symptoms, including pain, numbness, and tingling in the buttocks, hips, and legs. The peroneal nerve is one of the two branches of the sciatic nerve that supplies sensation and movement to the lower legs and feet. Peroneal neuropathy is a type of nerve damage that can happen anywhere along the peroneal nerve's course due to compression or irritation. In this chapter, we will discuss peroneal neuropathy in the context of PS, including its anatomy, causes, symptoms, diagnosis, and treatment options.

2   Anatomy

The sciatic nerve is the longest and largest peripheral nerve in the body. It is derived from the ventral rami of the L4–S3 spinal nerves. The nerve usually exits the pelvis via a single trunk through the greater sciatic foramen below the piriformis muscle, and courses in the posterior thigh compartment. This nerve consists of two divisions: the lateral division includes the common peroneal nerve fibers and the medial division is formed by the tibial nerve fibers (Preston and Shapiro 2013). Although the tibial and common peroneal nerve fibers are surrounded by a common epineural sheath, the tibial and peroneal fascicular groups are separated by connective tissue (Sladjana

G. G. Güleç (✉)
Istanbul, Turkey
e-mail: gamzegulgulec@gmail.com

K. M. Iyer (ed.), *Piriformis Syndrome*,
https://doi.org/10.1007/978-3-031-40736-9_16

et al. 2008). The nerve divides proximally into the tibial and common peroneal nerves at a variable level when it reaches the popliteal fossa (Fig. 1).

The lateral cutaneous nerve branch of the knee emerges first from the common peroneal nerve and provides a sensation to the lateral part of the knee. The nerve then wraps around the fibular neck and divides into superficial and deep segments (Preston and Shapiro 2013). The deep branch, which innervates the ankle and toe dorsiflexors and provides sensation to the area between the first and second toes. The superficial peroneal nerve innervates the muscles that evert the ankle and provides sensation to the middle and lower lateral calf, up to the level of the interphalangeal joint of 3 or 4 fingers on the dorsum of the foot (Preston and Shapiro 2013).

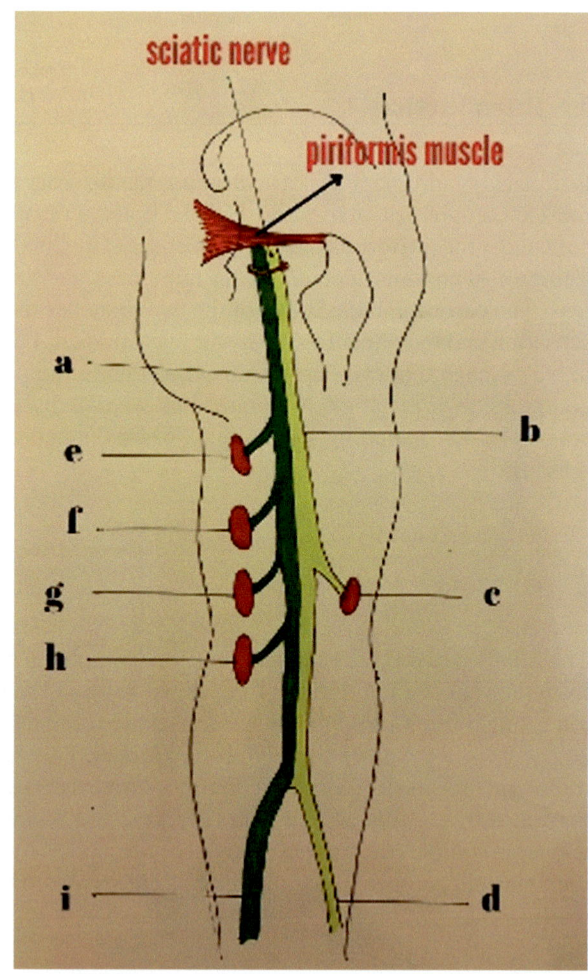

Fig. 1 Branches of the sciatic nerve and muscles innervated by the sciatic nerve in the thigh. Sciatic nerve exits the pelvis via a single trunk below the piriformis muscle. The nerve consists of the medial tibial and lateral peroneal fascicular groups which are separated by connective tissue. a) tibial branch of the sciatic nerve b) peroneal branch of sciatic nerve c) short head of biceps femoris d) common peroneal nerve e) semimembranosus f) semitendinosus g) long head of biceps femoris h) ischial part of adductor magnus I) tibial nerve

3 Peroneal Neuropathy in Piriformis Syndrome

Peroneal neuropathy usually presents with a drop foot and sensory disturbances on the lateral part of the calf and dorsum of the foot (Baima and Krivickas 2008). It most commonly occurs in the neck of the fibula where the nerve is very superficial and vulnerable to damage (Baima and Krivickas 2008). However, patients with lumbar plexopathy, L5 radiculopathy and sciatic neuropathy may show a similar pattern of numbness and weakness because the peroneal fibers are sensitive and primarily affected (Preston and Shapiro 2013). As with other injuries of the sciatic nerve in the gluteal region (such as fractures, dislocations or iatrogenic injuries), the peroneal fibers are the most susceptible to injury and prominently affected in PS. The reason for this is explained by the lateral localization of the nerve fibers, the larger size of the division and the tethering at the fibular head (Baima and Krivickas 2008). In addition, anatomical variations of the piriformis muscle and sciatic nerve are thought to be predisposed to the development of PS and affect its clinical presentation (Pećina 1979; Güleç et al. 2022). The compression of the sciatic nerve can result in damage or compression of the peroneal nerve branches, leading to motor and sensory deficits in the leg (Pećina 1979).

4 Diagnosis

The diagnosis of peroneal neuropathy in PS can be challenging, as the symptoms are similar to those of other conditions, such as peripheral neuropathy or lumbar radiculopathy. Diagnosis typically involves anamnesis, a thorough physical examination, nerve conduction studies, imaging studies such as magnetic resonance imaging (MRI) and diagnostic injection (Jankovic et al. 2013; Probst et al. 2019; Smith et al. 2006).

Peroneal neuropathy related to PS can present with various clinical findings. Patients may complain of toes constantly hitting the ground while walking and pain, numbness, tingling, or weakness in the foot and ankle, which may be exacerbated by longtime sitting (Hopayian and Danielyan 2018; Gulec et al. 2020; Yildirim et al. 2015; Aydemir et al. 2010; Moon et al. 2015). They may also experience difficulty dorsiflexing the foot or extending the toes, as well as a loss of sensation on the top of the foot (Gulec et al. 2020; Yildirim et al. 2015; Aydemir et al. 2010; Moon et al. 2015). Physical examination may reveal weakness of the muscles responsible for ankle dorsiflexion and toe extension, which are supplied by the peroneal nerve (Gulec et al. 2020; Yildirim et al. 2015; Aydemir et al. 2010; Moon et al. 2015). Deep palpation of the piriformis muscle is mostly painful (Hopayian and Danielyan 2018; Gulec et al. 2020; Yildirim et al. 2015). Patients may experience aggravation of symptoms with PS-specific maneuvers, such as the Freiberg test, Pace sign, Heel Contralateral Knee (HCLK) test, Flexion Adduction and Internal Rotation (FAİR) and Beatty tests (Jankovic et al. 2013; Probst et al. 2019; Hopayian and Danielyan

2018). The Straight Leg Raise (SLR) was found to be positive in 31% of the PS patients (Hopayian and Danielyan 2018). However, these clinical findings may also be positive in pathologies, such as facet syndrome, sacroiliac joint problems and lumbar disc herniation (Probst et al. 2019). Additionally, the sensitivity and specificity of PS-specific maneuvers are controversial (Jankovic et al. 2013; Probst et al. 2019).

MRI can provide useful information. Pelvic MRI may reveal piriformis muscle atrophy (Hettler 2006), muscle hypertrophy (Yildirim et al. 2015; Aydemir et al. 2010; Moon et al. 2015) or muscle asymmetry (Yildirim et al. 2015; Aydemir et al. 2010; Moon et al. 2015; Hettler 2006), perineural edema (Yildirim et al. 2015; Aydemir et al. 2010; Moon et al. 2015), space occupying lesions (such as endometriosis) (Hettler 2006), SN variants or fibrotic bands (Moon et al. 2015). Additionally, MRI may detect other structural abnormalities, such as a herniated disc or spinal stenosis, which may contribute to nerve compression. Overall, MRI findings can provide valuable information regarding the underlying cause of peroneal neuropathy and help guide treatment decisions. However, PS is mostly myofascial in origin, and MRI findings that explain the etiology should not be expected in every case (Jankovic et al. 2013).

Electrodiagnostic studies are most useful in ruling out peroneal neuropathy at the fibular head and other causes, such as lumbosacral radiculopathy and plexopathy. Electrodiagnostic studies are usually normal unless severe, longstanding compression has led to denervation of the muscle (Jankovic et al. 2013; Probst et al. 2019; Gulec et al. 2020). Electromyography (EMG) findings may show abnormalities in the peroneal nerve and the muscles it innervates (Yildirim et al. 2015; Aydemir et al. 2010; Moon et al. 2015; Hettler 2006). Specifically, EMG may detect decreased recruitment or firing of the muscles supplied by the peroneal nerve (Yildirim et al. 2015; Moon et al. 2015). Regardless of the suspected site of nerve compromise, examining the short head of the biceps femoris is important. EMG demonstrates membrane instability of the short head of the biceps femoris muscle in lesions proximal to the fibular head. Needle EMG of the paraspinal muscles is important to exclude the diagnosis of lumbar radiculopathy (Moon et al. 2015; Hettler 2006). However, it should not be forgotten that PS and lumbar radiculopathy can be seen together (Gulec et al. 2020).

The inability to establish diagnostic criteria for PS has created a need for alternative diagnostic methods. Local anesthetic (LA) injection into the PM is considered a reference diagnostic test (Jankovic et al. 2013; Probst et al. 2019; Smith et al. 2006; Gulec et al. 2020; Yildirim et al. 2015; Aydemir et al. 2010). More than 50% of post-injection pain relief and the inability to provoke pain with post-injection provocation tests are helpful in the diagnosis of PS (Smith et al. 2006; Niu et al. 2009). Due to the deep location of the piriformis muscle, its small size, and its closeness to neurovascular structures, it is recommended that the injection be done with the help of imaging (Jankovic et al. 2013; Probst et al. 2019). This will make the injection more reliable and accurate.

Ultrasound (US) seems to be superior to other imaging methods for guiding injections into the piriformis muscle because it is cheap, easy to get, has dynamic imaging, and can show blood vessels without contrast (Fig. 2).

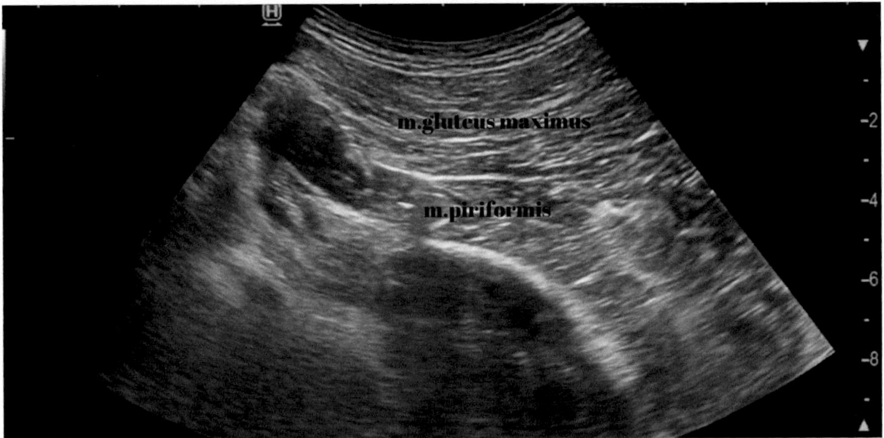

Fig. 2 Sonographic Evaluation of the Piriformis Muscle. The piriformis muscle was visualized in deep localization under the gluteus maximus muscle. Ultrasound imaging is a low-cost, easily accessible imaging technique. Dynamic imaging could be performed during the injection. This increases the safety and reliability of the injection

US also provides the opportunity to examine the course of the nerve. With careful examination and imaging with diagnostic US, sciatic nerve variations could be visualized in patients with PS (Güleç et al. 2022). In case of peroneal compression, enlargement of the nerve proximal to the site of compression, decreased echogenicity, and increased vascularity could be seen (Suk et al. 2013).

5   Treatment

Treatment of peroneal neuropathy in PS typically involves addressing the underlying cause of compression. Non-surgical treatment options may include physical therapy, LA, corticosteroid and Botulinum toxin type A injections (Jankovic et al. 2013; Probst et al. 2019). The injection of LA, steroids, and botulinum toxin A into the piriformis muscle can contribute to both diagnostic and therapeutic purposes (Smith et al. 2006). The muscular strength of dorsiflexors may significantly improve following injections if the sciatic nerve damage is not chronic and irreversible (Gulec et al. 2020; Yildirim et al. 2015; Aydemir et al. 2010). In chronic cases, improvement in neurological findings could not be obtained, but a relief in pain and paresthesia was mostly achieved (Moon et al. 2015; Hettler 2006). Physical therapy including the piriformis muscle stretching and strengthening the muscles of the lower extremity must be added to the treatment protocol (Gulec et al. 2020; Yildirim et al. 2015; Aydemir et al. 2010; Moon et al. 2015).

If conservative treatment fails and the symptoms become persistent and disabling, surgical intervention may be necessary to decompress the nerve (Jankovic et al. 2013;

Probst et al. 2019; Moon et al. 2015; Hettler 2006). Decompression of space occupying lesions (Hettler 2006), PM release (Moon et al. 2015) or tenotomy may resolve the symptoms. Complications such as hematoma, infection, involuntary internal rotation of the hip, or in-toeing gait could be observed, and the surgical results could not be satisfactory in every case (Probst et al. 2019; Moon et al. 2015; Indrekvam and Sudmann 2002).

In summary, peroneal neuropathy can occur in the context of PS because peroneal fibers are sensitive to compression as they pass through the muscles. PS should be considered in the differential diagnosis of patients with peroneal neuropathy. Unlike isolated peroneal neuropathy, these patients may complain of gluteal pain, in addition to numbness, tingling, weakness, and pain in the lower leg and foot. The symptoms are aggravated by long-term siting. Deep gluteal palpation was tender in most patients. Pelvic MRI can be used to confirm the diagnosis and exclude lumbar disc herniation. Electrodiagnostic studies are helpful for ruling out alternative diagnoses. A > 50% reduction in symptoms after intramuscular LA injection confirm diagnosis, indicating that peroneal neuropathy is due to PS. With proper management, most patients experience improvement in their symptoms and maintain good functional outcomes.

References

Aydemir K, Duman I, TugcuI,Ozgul A. Piriformis syndrome presenting with foot drop diagnosed with magnetic resonance Imaging: a case report. J Musculoskelet Pain. 2010;18(3):261–4.

Baima J, Krivickas L. Evaluation and treatment of peroneal neuropathy. Curr Rev Musculoskelet Med. 2008;1(2):147–53.

Güleç GG, Kurt Oktay KN, Aktaş İ, Yilmaz B. Visualizing anatomic variants of the sciatic nerve using diagnostic ultrasound during piriformis muscle injection: an example of 4 cases. J Chiropr Med. 2022;21(3):213–9.

Gulec GG, Aktaş İ, Ünlü Özkan F, Bayrak D. An unusual case of piriformis syndrome: peroneal neuropathy. Bosphorus Med J. 2020;7(2):63–6.

Hettler A, Bo¨hm J, Pretzsch M, von Salis-Soglio G (2006) Extragenital endometriosis leading to piriformis syndrome. Nervenarzt. 2006;77:474–7.

Hopayian K, Danielyan A. Four symptoms define the piriformis syndrome: an updated systematic review of its clinical features. Eur J Orthop Surg Traumatol. 2018;28:155–64.

Indrekvam K, Sudmann E. Piriformis muscle syndrome in 19 patients treated by tenotomy—a 1- to 16-year follow-up study. Int Orthop. 2002;26:101–3.

Jankovic D, Peng P, van Zundert A. Brief review: piriformis syndrome: etiology, diagnosis, and management. Can J Anaesth. 2013;60(10):1003–12.

Kirschner JS, Foye PM, Cole JL. Piriformis syndrome, diagnosis, and treatment. Muscle Nerve. 2009;40(1):10–8.

Moon HB, Nam KY, Kwon BS, Park JW, Ryu GH, Lee HJ, Kim CJ. Leg weakness caused by bilateral piriformis syndrome: a case report. Ann Rehabil Med. 2015;39(6):1042–6.

Niu C, Lai P, Fu T, Chen L, Chen W. Ruling out piriformis syndrome before diagnosing lumbar radiculopathy. Chang Gung Med J. 2009;32:182–7.

Pećina M. Contribution to the etiological explanation of the piriformis syndrome. Acta Anat (Basel). 1979;105(2):181–7.

Preston DC, Shapiro BE. Peroneal neuropathy. In: Preston DC, Shapiro BE, editors. Electromyography and neuromuscular disorders, 3rd ed. Saunders: 2013. p. 346–56.

Preston DC, Shapiro BE. Sciatic neuropathy. In: Preston DC, Shapiro BE, editors. Electromyography and neuromuscular disorders, 3rd ed. Saunders; 2013. p. 518–28.

Probst D, Stout A, Hunt D. Piriformis syndrome: a narrative review of the anatomy, diagnosis, and treatment. PM R. 2019;11(1):54–63.

Sladjana UZ, Ivan JD, Bratislav SD. Microanatomical structure of the human sciatic nerve. Surg Radiol Anat. 2008;30:619–26.

Smith J, Hurdle MF, Locketz AJ, Wisniewski SJ. Ultrasound-guided piriformis injection: technique description and verification. Arch Phys Med Rehabil. 2006;87:1664–7.

Suk JI, Walker FO, Cartwright MS. Ultrasonography of peripheral nerves. Curr Neurol Neurosci Rep. 2013;13(2):328.

Yildirim P, Guler T, Misirlioglu TO, Ozer T, Gunduz OH. A case of drop foot due to piriformis syndrome. Acta Neurol Belg. 2015;115(4):847–9.

Physiotherapy in Piriformis Syndrome

Sushumna Tiwarrii

1 Introduction

The piriformis muscle originates from the anterior surface of the sacrum and passes posterolaterally through the sciatic notch to insert into the upper border of the greater trochanter (Brukner 2002).

Piriformis syndrome is caused by macrotrauma to the buttocks, which is leading to soft tissue inflammation and nerve compression. Patients usually suffer from pain in the buttocks, low back which may be radiating, numbness, difficulty sitting comfortably, difficulty with walking, and while performing daily living activities (Kirschner 2009).

Piriformis syndrome is most misunderstood, and it is controversial, and often misdiagnosed and confused because this syndrome's symptoms are like many other conditions like low back pain, lumbar radiculopathy, primary sacral dysfunction, and sciatica. The therapist should understand the structure and function of the piriformis muscle and he is also able to identify how it relates to the sciatic nerve. A detailed approach to diagnosis requires a thorough musculoskeletal and neurological history, and physical assessment of the patient based on the clinical signs and symptoms of piriformis syndrome (https://jom.osteopathic.org/abstract/diagnosis-and-management-of-piriformis-syndrome-an-osteopathic-approach/). Physiotherapists focus mainly on stretching, modalities, and various exercises while treating piriformis syndrome.

S. Tiwarrii (✉)
MBA – Healthcare Management, San Jose, California, USA
e-mail: sushumna2020@gmail.com

    97
K. M. Iyer (ed.), *Piriformis Syndrome*,
https://doi.org/10.1007/978-3-031-40736-9_17

2 Physiotherapy Management

Special tests screen the piriformis muscle tightness, pain, and discomfort in the surrounding area. There are many special tests for piriformis syndrome.

- Piriformis test: The Patient should be in a side lying position by placing the involved leg on top. The patient should flex the involved hip to 60° with the knee flexed. Pain is elicited if there is tightness in the piriformis muscle. Buttock pain and sciatica may be experienced if piriformis pinches the sciatic nerve (Magee 2021).
- Pace sign (resisted abduction and external rotation of the thigh): In the pace test, the patient should be in a sitting position or supine lying position. The patient should abduct and externally rotate his hips against resistance applied by the examiner. Pain and weakness are felt by resisted abduction and external rotation of the hip. If there is a pain in the buttocks, the test is considered positive.
- Freiberg (forceful internal rotation of the extended thigh): The patient lies in the supine position with the thigh extended. Therapist should passively internally rotate the leg and the thigh. The test is positive if pain and weakness are noticed. Piriformis stretching and pressure placed on the sciatic nerve at the sacrospinous ligament causes pain.
- Fair test: During the test, the patient should be in a lying position with the injured leg on top. Passively flex the affected hip into 90° of flexion, horizontal adduction, and internal rotation. Reproduction of pain and tenderness at the buttocks is considered as a positive test for piriformis syndrome.
- Beatty's test: In this test, the patient should lie on the uninvolved side, he should lift and hold the superior knee around 4 inches off the table. Abduction here causes deep pain in the buttocks in piriformis syndrome patients but back and leg pain in lumbar disc disease individuals (Hicks 2022).
- SLR Test or League's test: While performing the straight leg raising test or League's test, the Patient should lie in the supine position. The therapist will lift the extended leg of a patient. This test clinically demonstrates lumbosacral radicular irritation. The test is positive when the patient experiences pain along the course of lumbar root distribution (Ojha 2017).

3 Physical Therapy Interventions

Physiotherapists combine exercises with massage to get quick relief. Massage helps in improving blood circulation, which creates better healing in the affected area. Massage also reduces stress and relaxes tight muscles. Tight muscles sometimes get knotted up into painful nodules. Massage therapy can stretch and loosen up the muscle. Deep tissue massage, myofascial release, and active release techniques may be applied at the buttock and thigh areas during exercise sessions (https://www.spine-health.com/blog/massage-ease-sciatica-pain).

Electrotherapy Modalities: Electrotherapy uses electrical stimulation to improve muscle function, to reduce pain, and promote tissue healing. Various electrotherapy modalities may be used to treat signs and symptoms of piriformis syndrome. Ultrasound, TENS, and LASER are a few of them.

Ultrasound: Use 2.0–2.5 W/cm^2, for 10–14 min. Ultrasound gel was applied around the piriformis muscle. Ultrasound helps to break down myofascial triggers in the muscle. Piriformis stretching is often performed after the application of ultrasound therapy (Leong 2020).

Transcutaneous electric nerve stimulation (TENS) is a portable and inexpensive therapeutic device that can help to block pain, decrease muscle strain and spasms.

Laser treatment uses focussed light to reduce pain and inflammation and promotes healing. Laser therapy efficacy varies from patient to patient. Laser rays can penetrate deeply and stimulate cell repair and helps in the healing process of piriformis muscle (Ojha 2017).

4 Hot Packs/Cold Packs

A simple home remedy to reduce pain in the buttocks is to apply a cold pack or heating pad over the affected area. To reduce pain, apply hot packs or cold packs for at least 10 min before stretching the piriformis muscle.

Heat therapy improves blood circulation by dilating blood vessels. Improving circulation to the affected part will reduce stiffness, calm painful muscle spasms, and improves the healing process. Hot water bottles, hot towels, heat wraps, and electric heat pads can be used for 15 min approximately. Overuse of heat packs may damage skin and produce burns and scales.

Cold therapy or ice massage helps to decrease circulation and blood flow by constricting the blood vessels. Therefore, pain, inflammation, and swelling reduce through a numbing effect. Ice packs, cold wraps, or gel packs can be applied for 15 min approximately. Overuse of ice packs damages the skin, superficial nerves, and frostbite may be seen (https://www.spine-health.com/conditions/sciatica/cold-and-heat-therapy-sciatica).

Simple piriformis muscle stretching is encouraged after the application of packs. These stretches help to relieve pain. Apply heat before stretching to warm the piriformis and use an ice pack after the piriformis stretch to soothe activity-related flare-ups.

5 Piriformis Stretching

While stretching the piriformis muscle, apply pressure at the inferior border of the muscle, and while pressing, pressure is applied tangentially and do not press downward because the sciatic nerve may compress against the gamellus superior tendinious edge. Muscle grip gets weak when applying pressure on the nerve and pain gets relieved at piriformis syndrome.

The Piriformis muscle is also stretched in a FAIR position. The lumbosacral corset is used while the patient lying in the supine position. When the patient is in the supine position, the Hip is flexed, adducted, and medially rotated. Now the patient gets his involved side foot across and over the uninvolved side knee. Physiotherapist performs Muscle Energy Technique where the patient abducts his leg against mild resistance for 5 s with 5 repetitions.

6 Piriformis One Stretch/Supine Piriformis Stretch

In supine lying position, the patient should pull the knee towards his shoulder. Hold for 30 s until the stretch is felt and do the same with the other leg (Fig. 1). Repeat it for three times, twice a day (https://proceedings.ums.ac.id/index.php/apc/article/download/116/117/124).

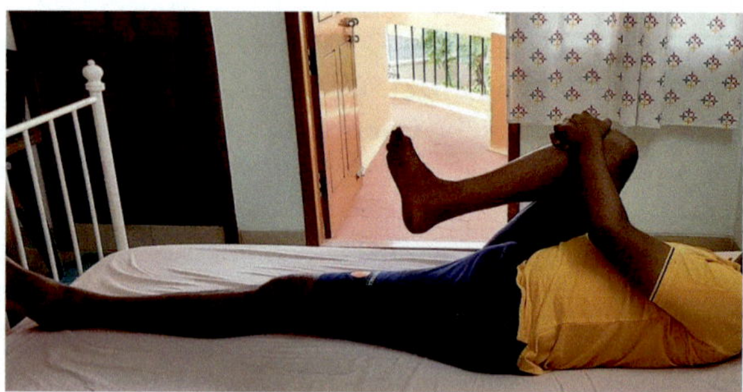

Fig. 1 Supine piriformis stretch

Fig. 2 Crossbody piriformis stretch

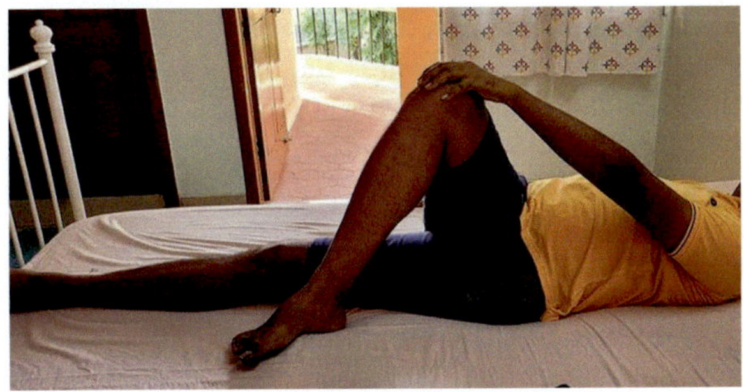

7 Piriformis Two Stretch/Crossbody Piriformis Stretch (Fig. 2)

In supine lying position, the patient should raise the involved leg and place the uninvolved foot across the body. The patient should place his opposite side hand to pull the involved knee towards the floor. Gently pull the knee until a proper stretch is felt around the buttock's region. Hold the stretch for 30 s and come back to normal position. The aim is to perform three sets on each side (https://proceedings.ums.ac. id/index.php/apc/article/download/116/117/124).

8 Piriformis Three Stretch/Ankle Over Knee Stretch/Knee to Chest Stretch (Fig. 3)

The patient should be in a supine lying position with both knees bent. Keep the ankle on the opposite side of the knee.

Fig. 3 Knee to chest stretch

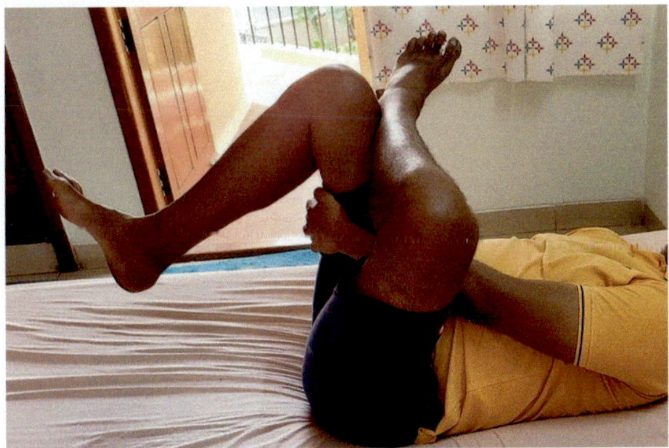

Both hands and placed posterior to the thigh on the lower leg behind your opposite knee. Pull the thigh towards the chest until the patient feels a stretch around the buttocks. Hold the stretch for 30 s or less based on the patient tolerance level. Three stretches should be performed on each side (https://proceedings.ums.ac.id/index.php/apc/article/download/116/117/124).

9   Seated Piriformis Stretch

The patient should sit on a chair and cross one foot over the opposite knee (Figs. 4 and 5) Pull the top knee across to the opposite side shoulder and the foot should be rested on the bottom knee. Hold for 30 s. Based on the patient's tolerance, he can increase the stretch by drawing the knee further. He can perform the exercise while sitting on the floor too if he is not comfortable in the chair (Clayton 2016).

Fig. 4 Seated piriformis stretch

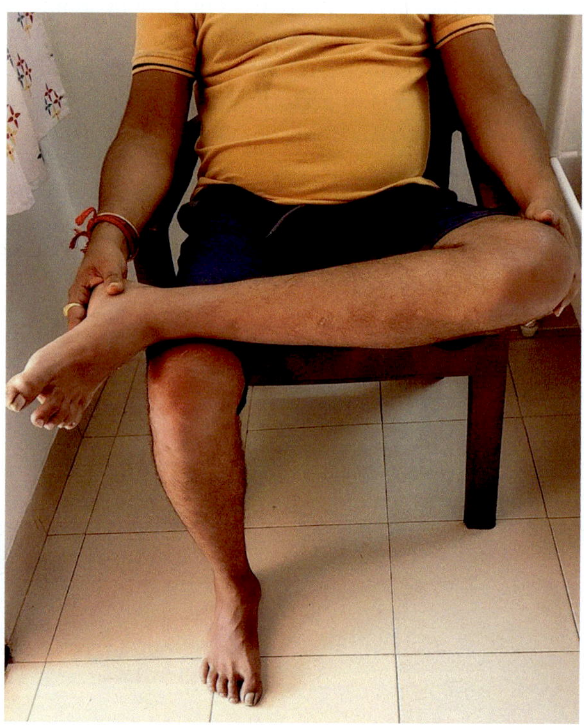

Fig. 5 Seated piriformis
stretch

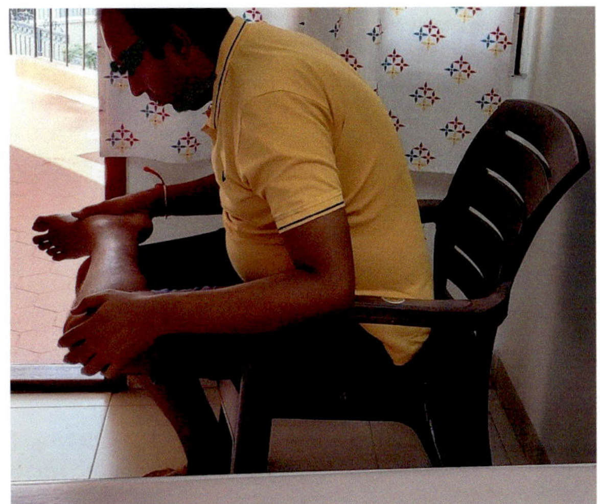

10   Standing Piriformis Stretch (Fig. 6)

The patient can stand facing a table where he can place one leg up. He should slightly
lean forward and he can use the table for balancing himself. He should lean forward
and feel his piriformis muscle stretch. Hold it for 30 s. He can progress to mini squat
further.

Fig. 6 Standing piriformis
stretch

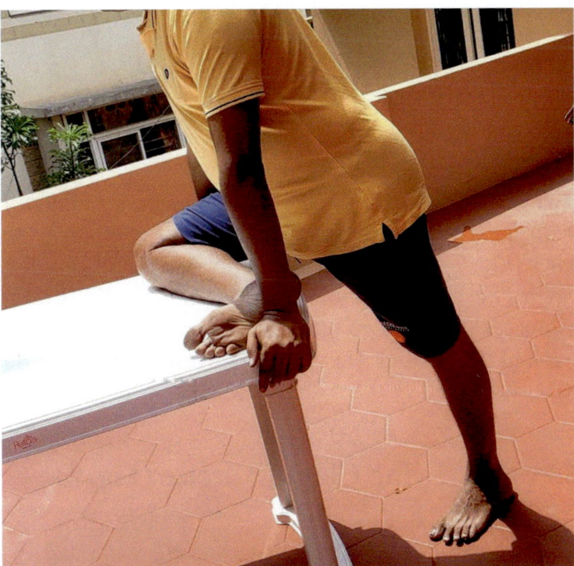

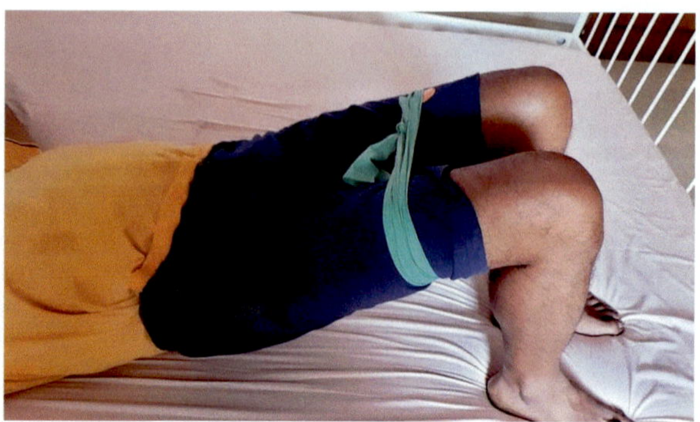

Fig. 7 Bridge with
TheraBand (Fig. 7)

The purpose of this stretching is to improve the length of the piriformis muscle which is shortened and decrease pressure on the sciatic nerve (Ahmad Siraj 2022).

11 Strengthening Exercises

Strengthening exercises should focus on the piriformis and other hip muscles like hip abductors, extensors, external rotators, and movement re-education. This is crucial for building muscle strength and developing resilience in the hip. The patient will work on his non-weight-bearing exercises, weight-bearing exercises, and Dynamic and ballistic training. Patients may be advised to reduce the amount of hip adduction and internal rotation during the weight-bearing program.

12 Bridge

The bridge position should be performed initially without the Thera band and later with the Thera band wrapped around the patient's thighs near the proximal to the knee (Fig. 7). The patient raises his pelvis and simultaneously abducts and externally rotates his hips. Hold this position for 5 s initially and work up to 30 s. He should not allow his thighs to go into adduction and internal rotation while lowering his pelvis back to the ground. He should perform three times daily (Tonley 2010).

13 Side-Lying Clam Exercise (Fig. 8)

In the beginning, perform this exercise without any resistance, with hip and knee flexed at 45°, and keep feet together. The patient should elevate his knee up and back, by doing hip abduction and external rotation. After he can perform 10–15 few

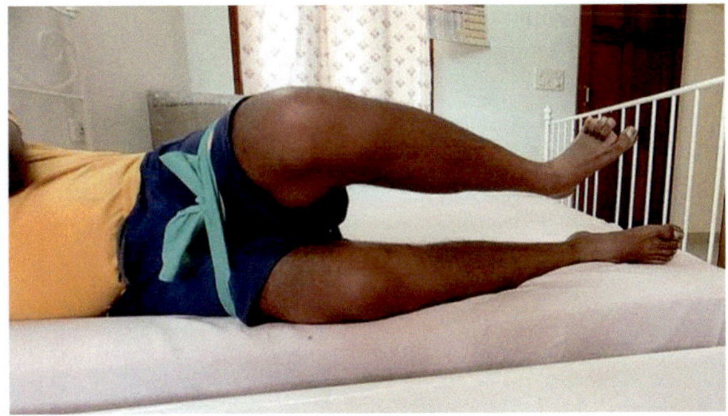

Fig. 8 Side lying clam with resistance (Fig. 8)

clam exercises, progress with TheraBand wrapped around the thigh proximal to the knee. Later, repeat with the opposite leg. Try to complete 3 sets of repetitions a day.

Start with double-limb weight-bearing exercises and then progress to single-limb weight-bearing exercises which improve the demands of hip muscles.

14   Squat (Fig. 9)

The patient should perform a squat initially at 45° depth of hip and knee flexion and then progress to 75°. Later, squat with Thera band resistance applied around the thighs close to the proximal area of the knees.

The patient should progress to a side-stepping exercise with Thera-band. The patient should start with squats of 45° of hip and knee flexion, and he should take steps to the left and right by abducting and laterally rotating his hips (Fig. 10). He should control his hip in frontal and transverse planes and his trunk should be maintained straight while performing the exercise (Tonley 2010).

15   Lunges and Jumps

Complete the exercises like lunges and squats which may strengthen all related muscle groups including the piriformis, weak hamstrings, gluteus, and hips.

As the patient gets pain-free, if he experiences normal strength, the patient should progress to perform different types of lunges such as forward lunge (Fig. 11), lunge at 45°, double limb jumps with double limb landing position with a deep squat (Fig. 12) and double limb jump/right and left single limb landings. He should perform single-limb landings without doing excess hip adduction and internal rotation (Tonley 2010).

Fig. 9 Squat with the theraband resistance

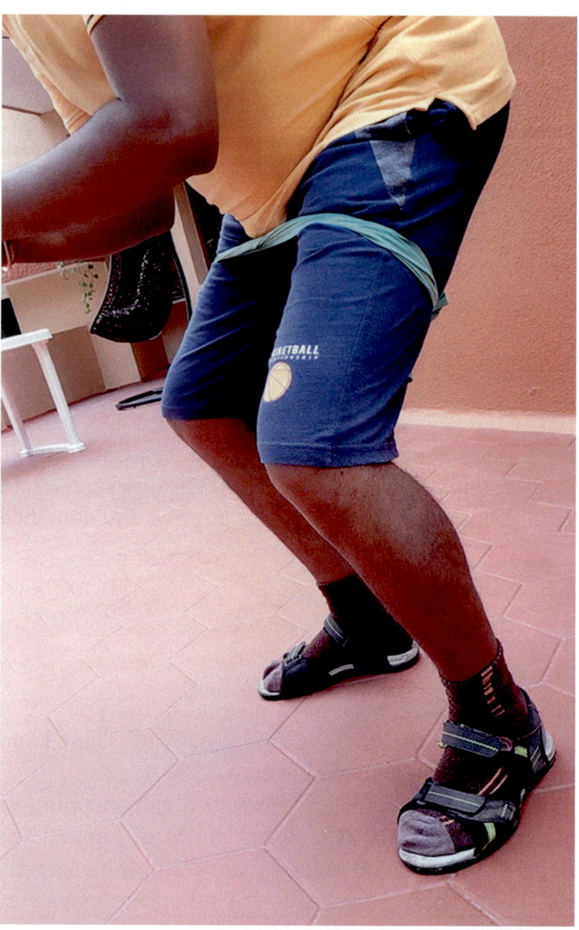

Fig. 10 Sidestep with the thera-band resistance

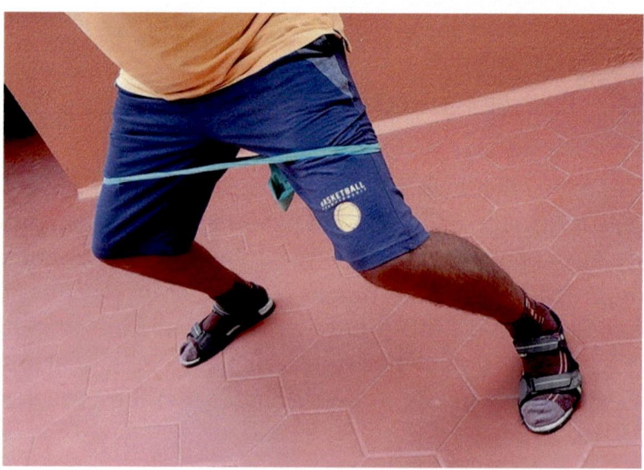

Fig. 11 Forward lunge

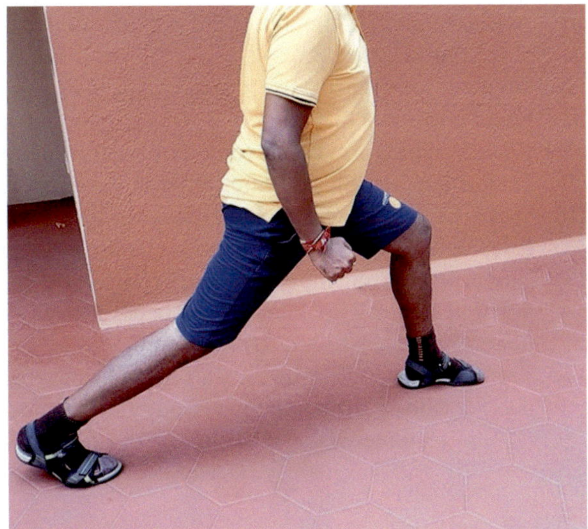

Fig. 12 Double limb Jump/
lands position

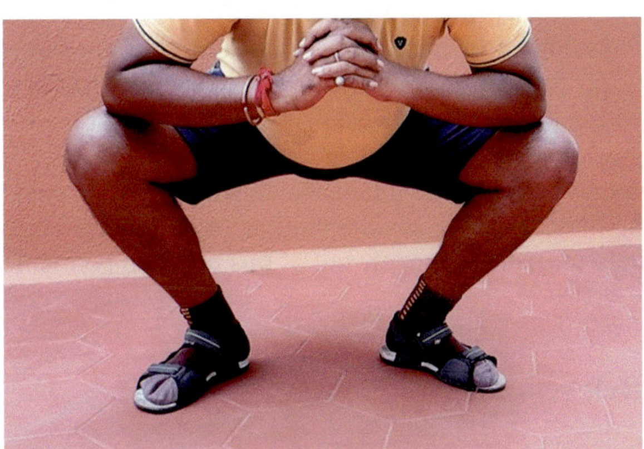

16 Things to "Do" and to "Avoid" in Piriformis Syndrome Patients

1. Avoid sitting for a long period of time; take a break and walk every 20 min.
2. To avoid the recurrence of the piriformis syndrome, daily exercises, and stretching are important.
3. Avoid sitting in a soft chair or low chair. If your knees are higher than your hips, that may lead to pressure on the piriformis and result in piriformis tightness.
4. Patient should sit on a cushion. This may help in cushioning the effect on the buttocks and help to raise his hips.

5. Avoid running, hiking up, avoid activities that could compress the sciatic nerve at the buttock region.
6. Do piriformis muscle exercises regularly, but always stretch the muscle first.
7. Good posture is maintained in sitting, standing, and driving.
8. Recurrent pain can be prevented by performing exercises consistently.
9. Performing aerobic activities at least 30 min, 5 times per week is essential.
10. Water exercises are also beneficial. This may be encouraged if a patient feels severe pain when he is performing land-based exercises.
11. Lift an object from the ground only by bending the knees and being in a squatting position to pick it up. Don't lift by bending over. Avoid twisting your body while doing the activity.
12. Ergonomic standing desks and ergonomic chairs are good investments for people who work on their computers for a long time. Sitting in the wrong posture may increase the likelihood of piriformis tightness (Hicks 2022).

17 Conclusion

Physiotherapy treatment plays a huge role in piriformis syndrome. The prognosis of piriformis syndrome patients is excellent. Patients will become symptoms free within the first three weeks of their physiotherapy treatment program. If piriformis syndrome is untreated, that may lead to poor quality of life. Taking care of things to do and avoiding the things which will aggravate pain is an essential step to be taken by these patients. Maintaining aerobic and stretching activities will tremendously help the patient to come out of this problem permanently (Hicks 2022).

References

Ahmad Siraj SDR. Physiotherapy for piriformis syndrome using sciatic nerve mobilization and piriformis release. Cureus 2022;14(12):e32952. https://doi.org/10.7759/cureus.32952. Cited 30 Apr 2023.

Brukner PKK. Clinical sports medicine. London: McGraw-Hill Publishing; 2002.

Clayton P. Sacroiliac joint dysfunction and piriformis syndrome: the complete guide for physical therapists. Chichester, England: Lotus Publishing; 2016.

Cooper G. How massage can ease sciatic pain. Spine-Health. https://www.spine-health.com/blog/massage-ease-sciatica-pain. Cited 30 Apr 2023.

Cooper G. Cold and heat therapy for sciatica Spine-Health. https://www.spine-health.com/conditions/sciatica/cold-and-heat-therapy-sciatica. Cited 30 Apr 2023.

Diagnosis and management of piriformis syndrome: an osteopathic approach. J Osteopathic Med. 2021. https://jom.osteopathic.org/abstract/diagnosis-and-management-of-piriformis-syndrome-an-osteopathic-approach/. Cited 2023 Apr 30.

Hicks BL, Lam JC, Varacallo M. Piriformis Syndrome. StatPearls Publishing; 2022.

Kirschner JS, Foye PM, Cole JL. Piriformis syndrome, diagnosis and treatment. Muscle Nerve. 2009;40(1):10–8. https://pubmed.ncbi.nlm.nih.gov/19466717/. Cited 30 Apr 2023.

Leong M-KHP. Piriformis syndrome as the only initial manifestation of septic sacroiliac osteomyelitis. Clin Med. 2020;20(3):e18–9. https://www.researchgate.net/publication/318318 389_Pr

Magee DJ. Orthopedic physical assessment, 2021st ed.

Ojha SJC. To find the Efficacy of Therapeutic Laser for Piriformis Syndrome. J Mahatma Gandhi Univ Med Sci Technol. 2017;2(1):14–7. https://doi.org/10.5005/jp-journals-10057-0024

Tonley JC YSKRDJFSPC. Treatment of an individual with piriformis syndrome focusing on hip muscle strengthening and movement reeducation. A case report. J Orthop Sports Phys Ther. 2010;40(2):103–11. https://doi.org/10.2519/jospt.2010.3108

Yani JAKKSKTJSURK. The effect of self stretching on pain levels due to piriformis syndrome at teras health center, boyolali district. Ums.ac.id. https://proceedings.ums.ac.id/index.php/apc/art icle/download/116/117/124. Cited 30 Apr 2023.

Treatment of Piriformis Syndrome

K. Mohan Iyer

It may be divided into Conservative or Surgical treatments.

1 Nonoperative/Conservative

Treatment for piriformis syndrome begins with nonoperative modalities such as:

1. Oral analgesics (e.g. NSAIDs—ibuprofin, muscle relaxants, and gabapentin—Gabapentin mutes the pain signal from the sciatic nerve.)
2. Physical therapy: Regimens include nerve stretches

   (a) Knees to chest;
   (b) Cobra or modified cobra;
   (c) Seated hip stretch;
   (d) Standing hamstring stretch;
   (e) Seated spinal twist;
   (f) Knee to opposite shoulder;
   (g) Reclining pigeon pose;
   (h) Groin and long adductor muscle stretch, isometric exercises, gluteal muscle strengthening

3. Injections: The piriformis muscle may become irritated, swollen and tight due to injury resulting in twitching when It presses on the nearby sciatic nerve resulting in hip and buttock pain which may extend down the leg.During this an injection which is a combination of anesthetic (lidocaine or bupivacaine) and steroid (cortisone, Kenalog or dexamethasone) is injected in and around the piriformis muscle when the local anesthetic gives immediate relief and the steroid provides

K. Mohan Iyer (✉)
University of Bangalore, Bangalore, India
e-mail: kmiyer28@hotmail.com

K. M. Iyer (ed.), *Piriformis Syndrome*,
https://doi.org/10.1007/978-3-031-40736-9_18

a long-term relief decreasing the swelling and thereby decreases the pressure on the nerves resulting in relief from pain allowing the muscle to heal, aided by physiotherapy. This is usually done by aseptic precaution under an X-ray control throughout the procedure. This procedure takes about 3 weeks to heal with muscle relaxants. Certain musculoskeletal radiologists also use ultrasound to diagnose and treat piriformis syndrome to precisely guide injections.

Certain complications must be kept in mind such as pain, nerve injury, increased pain or allergic reaction to the medication used.

A piriformis injection is an injection of a long-lasting steroid into the piriformis muscle of buttock. This steroid medication injected will help decrase the inflammation and/or swelling around the nerves that pass near or through the piriformis muscle. This may by an ultrasound-guided trigger point injection for piriformis syndrome. The Piriformis Muscle Injection is an injection of local anesthetic with steroids into the piriformis muscle. This technique can be helpful to patients presenting with piriformis syndrome refractory to NSAIDS both in diagnosis and treatment.

The use of Botox for injections in patients with piriformis syndrome has shown positive results. It has a difficult access of the needle for deep location, the small size of the muscle, and the proximity to neurovascular structures. Ultrasound guidance is easy to use and painless and several studies describe its use during BoNT-A administration in Piriformis muscle syndrome (PMS)

2 Surgical Treatment

1. Using the diagnostic procedure involved a detailed physical examination, including a palpation test for tenderness over the origin (sacroiliac joint) or insertion of the short external rotators behind the trochanter (Fig. 1).

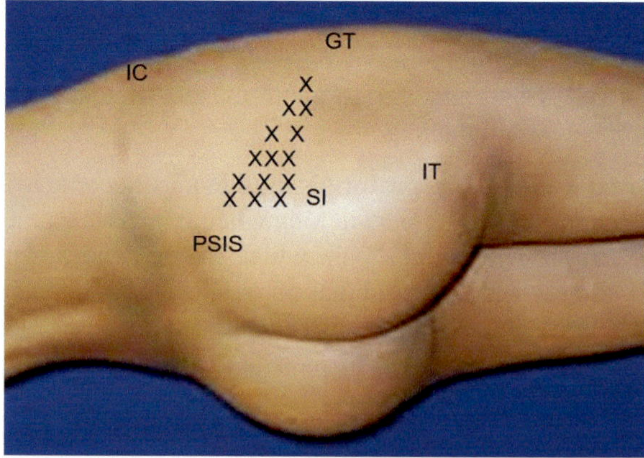

Fig. 1 Detailed physical examination: *Courtesy* Figure reproduced with the kind permission of Dr. Soo Hwan Kang, MD. Department of Orthopaedic Surgery, St. Paul's Hospital, College of Medicine, The Catholic University of Korea, 180 Wangsan-ro, Dongdaemun-gu, Seoul 02559, Korea

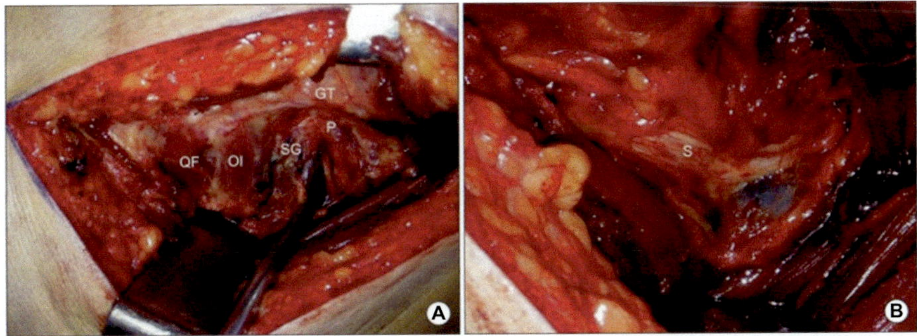

Fig. 2 **A, B** *Courtesy* Figure reproduced with the kind permission of Dr. Soo Hwan Kang, MD. Department of Orthopaedic Surgery, St. Paul's Hospital, College of Medicine, The Catholic University of Korea, 180 Wangsan-ro, Dongdaemun-gu, Seoul 02559, Korea

With the patient In the lateral decubitus position, using a curvilinear incision the gluteas maximus is separated by blunt dissextion in the direction of its fibres to locate the insertion of the piriformis into the posterior aspect of the greater trochanter which is above the insertion of the obturator internus tendon as seen in the Fig. 2a, b. Neurolysis around the sciatic nerve into the sciatic notch was performed in two cases of a severely adherent sciatic nerve. Severely dilated and engorged epineurial vessels were found in two cases with intractable sciatica as seen in the Fig. 5b.

2. Resection the piriformis muscle with/without neurolysis of the sciatic nerve

Details: Lateral decubitus position- curvilinear skin incision over the greater trochanter-through gluteus maximus- piriformis muscle is inserted into the posterior aspect of the greater trochanter as tendinous nature is identified above the obturator internus tendon-then the sciatic nerve was explored and found to pass anteriorly to the piriformis muscle- additionally, divide the tight piriformis tendon at the insertion site at its tendinous portion—proximal portion of the muscle is retracted when the leg was internally rotated after its division-then do a neurolysis around the sciatic nerve into the sciatic notch-postop pain is relieved by the use of a cane to relieve pain from the gluteal muscle repair. They had concluded that the piriformis muscle with/ without neurolysis of the sciatic nerve in patients who had intractable sciatica despite conservative treatment at least for 3 months and that it is a good treatment option in patients with refractory sciatica despite appropriate conservative treatments.

3. Endoscopic decompression of the sciatic nerve appears useful in improving function and diminishing hip pain in sciatic nerve entrapment/DGS.
4. They described 2 cases of piriformis syndrome caused by a rare type C sciatic nerve variation that were surgically treated using the transgluteal approach. A rare "C" type sciatic nerve variation was observed on the affected side under magnetic resonance imaging. Transgluteal sciatic nerve decompression provided significant pain relief.
5. Piriformis resection can be a feasible option for intractable piriformis syndrome.

6. Sciatica of nondisc origin and piriformis syndrome: diagnosis by magnetic resonance neurography and interventional magnetic resonance imaging with outcome study of resulting treatment.

This is reserved in refractory cases after exhausting nonoperative modalities and a 2005 study reported surgical outcomes in 64 patients managed with surgical intervention for refractory symptoms: showed:

(a) 82% reported initial improvement in their clinical status.
(b) 76% had long-term positive outcomes in the long run.
(c) 92% of those treated with surgery returned to work or presurgical baseline activity levels within 2 weeks of the surgery.

7. A Minimally Invasive Surgical Approach.

A minimally invasive approach utilizing a 6 cm skin incision is made posterior to the greater trochanter. The patient is positioned in the lateral decubitus position with the operative side upwards and the other knee flexed to 90° (Fig. 3).

An intermuscular plane was developed until the insertion of the piriformis tendon into the medial aspect of the greater trochanter was identified (Fig. 4).

The deep fascia over the gluteus maximus muscle (https://www.sciencedirect.com/topics/medicine-and-dentistry/gluteus-maximus-muscle)is divided longitudinally. An intermuscular plane was developed until the insertion of the piriformis tendon into the medial aspect of the greater trochanter was identified Fig. 2 *Courtesy* Figure reproduced with the kind permission of Adrian Kelly, Department of Neurosurgery, Dr. George Mukhari Academic Hospital, Sefako Makgatho Health Sciences University, Pretoria, South Africa.

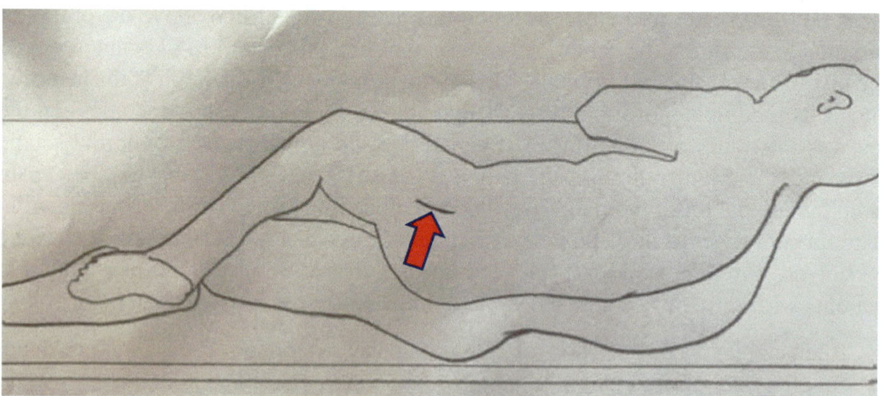

Fig. 3 Intra-operative sketch of patient positioning in the lateral position with the left side up, and the left knee flexed to 90°. The proposed minimally invasive 6 cm incision posterior to the left *greater trochanter* (https://www.sciencedirect.com/topics/medicine-and-dentistry/greater-trochanter) (red arrow) is also marked. *Courtesy* Figure reproduced with the kind permission of Adrian Kelly, Department of Neurosurgery, Dr. George Mukhari Academic Hospital, Sefako Makgatho Health Sciences University, Pretoria, South Africa

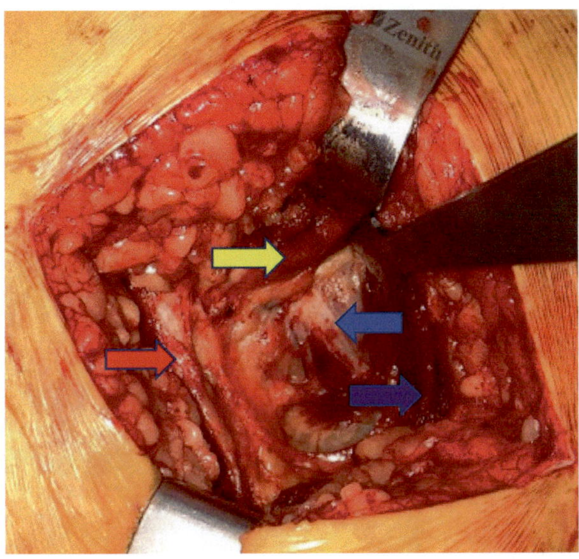

Fig. 4 An intra-operative photograph showing the 6 cm *skin incision* (https://www.sciencedirect.com/topics/medicine-and-dentistry/skin-incision) posterior to the left *greater trochanter* (https://www.sciencedirect.com/topics/medicine-and-dentistry/greater-trochanter) (deep to yellow arrow). The deep fascia (red arrow) over the *gluteus maximus muscle* (https://www.sciencedirect.com/topics/medicine-and-dentistry/gluteus-maximus-muscle) (purple arrow) has been divided, and the *gluteus muscle* (https://www.sciencedirect.com/topics/medicine-and-dentistry/gluteus-muscle) split longitudinally, to show the glistening bursa (blue arrow) over the piriformis tendon

Fig. 5 Patient diagram showing a posterior view of the anatomical relationship between the left piriformis muscle (red arrow) with the inflamed left *sciatic nerve* (https://www.sciencedirect.com/topics/medicine-and-dentistry/sciatic-nerve) (yellow arrow), emerging from beneath the left piriformis muscle, in relation to the bony pelvis. (*Courtesy* Figure reproduced with the kind permission of Adrian Kelly, Department of Neurosurgery, Dr. George Mukhari Academic Hospital, Sefako Makgatho Health Sciences University, Pretoria, South Africa)

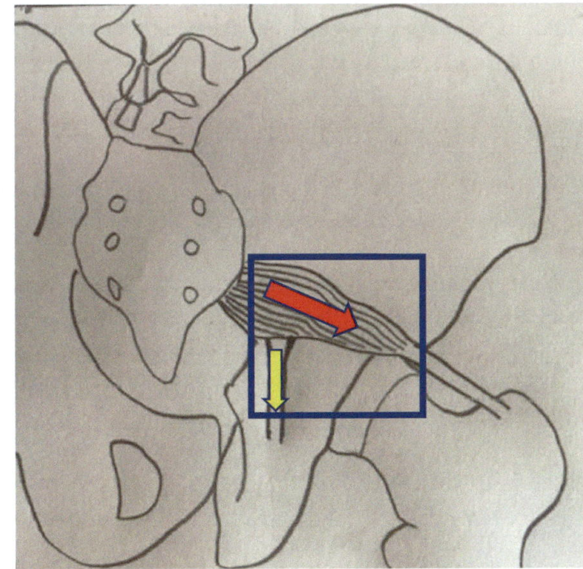

Fig. 6 An intra-operative photograph of the piriformis tendon (blue arrow) being lifted, post being dissected free

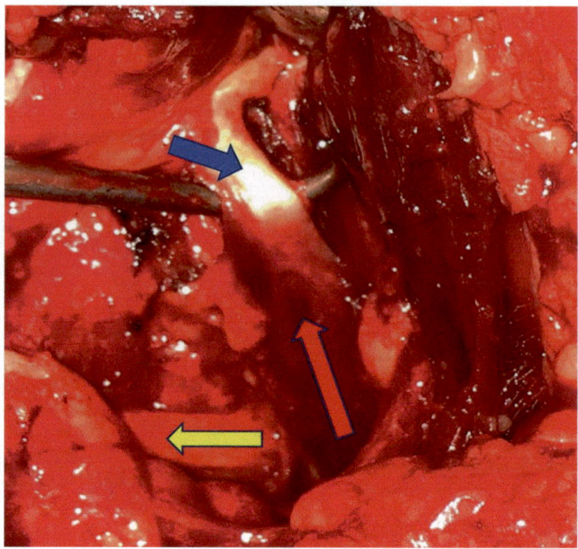

The compressed sciatic nerve was exposed diving deep to the piriformis tendon and was noted to be swollen and erythematous (Figs. 5 and 6).

The *sciatic nerve* (https://www.sciencedirect.com/topics/medicine-and-dentistry/sciatic-nerve) (yellow arrow) can be seen swollen and erythematous emerging from beneath the left piriformis muscle belly (red arrow) (*Courtesy* Fig. 7 reproduced with the kind permission of Adrian Kelly, Department of Neurosurgery, Dr. George Mukhari Academic Hospital, Sefako Makgatho Health Sciences University, Pretoria, South Africa).

This minimally invasive technique for treating piriformis syndrome is an effective treatment for this patient population. The positive results seen utilizing the novel integration of pre-operative trigger point localization coupled with intraoperative neuromonitoring make this surgical approach an attractive option.

Piriformis syndrome resolves quickly with lifestyle changes and simple treatments.

Numerous patients with piriformis syndrome will show symptomatic improvement after treatment with local trigger-point injection. When this is combined with rehabilitation exercises, the recurrences are rare.

Patients ungoing surgery for the release of adhesions and scars may take a few months to return to normal.

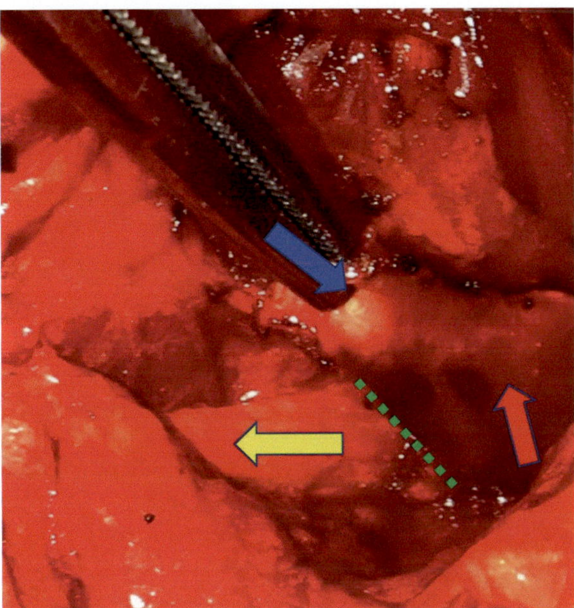

Fig. 7 An intra-operative photograph of the completely transected left piriformis tendon still being grasped with Alice forceps (blue arrow). Now that the tendon has been completely transected the left piriformis muscle is no longer under tension and has assumed a more globular shape (red arrow), relieving compression on the sciatic nerve (yellow arrow). A *neurolysis* (https://www.sci encedirect.com/topics/medicine-and-dentistry/neurolysis) comprising the dividing of fibrous adhesions in the interval (green dotted line) between the left piriformis muscle and left sciatic nerve has also been performed. *Courtesy* Figure reproduced with the kind permission of Adrian Kelly, Department of Neurosurgery, Dr. George Mukhari Academic Hospital, Sefako Makgatho Health Sciences University, Pretoria, South Africa

Complications with Prognosis

K. Mohan Iyer

1 Complications

Life-threatening complications include bacteraemia, which may lead to a poor outcome. Pelvic osteomyelitis is rare in adults, but it is associated with high morbidity and mortality.

Fever and severe pain. However, the pain may be poorly localised or accompanied by other non-specific symptoms. Piriformis syndrome due to sciatic nerve entrapment at the level of the ischial tuberosity may have sciatica-like pain in the gluteal region which is characterized as shooting, burning, or aching down the back of the leg. In addition, numbness in the buttocks and tingling sensations along the distribution of the sciatic nerve.

Complications related to surgery include: Nerve injury, Sciatic nerve injury is the most common, Infection and bleeding.

2 Prognosis

The prognosis is good in some cases once the piriformis sydnrome has been treated and they can lead a normal life. But in some cases the exercises need to be modified in order to reduce recurrence. Though control of pain by muscle relaxants, and anti-inflammatory drugs is beneficial, the patient may benefit from physical therapy for a longer while, piriformis syndrome is a soft tissue condition and may be diagnosed late may have a tendency to become chronic if not treated fully. Usually the response to local trigger-point injection is excellent with recurrences being uncommon and

K. Mohan Iyer (✉)
University of Bangalore, Bangalore, India
e-mail: kmiyer28@hotmail.com

K. M. Iyer (ed.), *Piriformis Syndrome*,
https://doi.org/10.1007/978-3-031-40736-9_19

athletes with piriformis syndrome show a pain-free range of movements with sufficient strength of the affected side to perform their sport-specific activities without discomfort.

If diagnosed piriformis syndrome early and the underlying cause is treated, the prognosis usually is good. However; piriformis syndrome in some people is diagnosed later in the disease. A later diagnosis has a less favorable prognosis if the disease has become chronic.

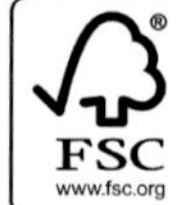
MIX
Papier aus verantwortungsvollen Quellen
Paper from responsible sources
FSC® C105338

If you have any concerns about our products,
you can contact us on
ProductSafety@springernature.com

In case Publisher is established outside the EU,
the EU authorized representative is:
Springer Nature Customer Service Center GmbH
Europaplatz 3, 69115 Heidelberg, Germany

Printed by Libri Plureos GmbH
in Hamburg, Germany